D1520209

Cerebral MR Perfusion Imaging

Principles and Current Applications

Cerebral MR Perfusion Imaging

Principles and Current Applications

A. Gregory Sorensen · Peter Reimer

215 Illustrations
6 Tables

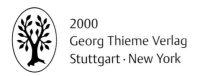

2000
Georg Thieme Verlag
Stuttgart · New York

A. Gregory Sorensen, M.D.
MGH-NMR Center
Building 149, 13th Street
MA 02129 Charlestown
USA

Priv.-Doz. Dr. Peter Reimer
Direktor des Zentralinstituts
für Bildgebende Diagnostik
Städtisches Klinikum Karlsruhe
Moltkestraße 90
76133 Karlsruhe
Germany

Library of Congress
Cataloging-in-Publication Data applied for

Die Deutsche Bibliothek – CIP-Einheitsaufnahme

Sorensen, A. Gregory:
Cerebral MR perfusion imaging : principles
and current applications / A. Gregory Sorensen ;
Peter Reimer. – Stuttgart ; New York :
Thieme, 2000

© 2000 Georg Thieme Verlag,
Rüdigerstrasse 14, 70469 Stuttgart,
Germany
Thieme New York, 333 Seventh Avenue
New York, NY 10001, USA

© 2000 Schering Aktiengesellschaft, Berlin

Printed in Germany

Graphics: Ziegler + Müller, Kirchentellinsfurt
Typesetting: Ziegler + Müller, Kirchentellinsfurt
Printing: Grammlich, Pliezhausen
Bookbinding: Heinr. Koch, Tübingen

ISBN 3-13-105401-8 (GTV)
ISBN 0-86577-925-2 (TNY)

2 3 4 5 6

Important Note: Medicine is an ever-changing science undergoing continual development. Research and clinical experience are continually expanding our knowledge, in particular our knowledge of proper treatment and drug therapy. Insofar as this book mentions any dosage or application, readers may rest assured that the authors, editors, and publishers have made every effort to ensure that such references are in accordance with **the state of knowledge at the time of production of the book.**

Nevertheless, this does not involve, imply, or express any guarantee or responsibility on the part of the publishers in respect to any dosage instructions and forms of applications stated in the book. **Every user is requested** to examine carefully the manufacturers' leaflets accompanying each drug and to check, if necessary in consultation with a physician or specialist, whether the dosage schedules mentioned therein or the contraindications stated by the manufacturers differ from the statements made in the present book. Such examination is particularly important with drugs that are either rarely used or have been newly released on the market. **Every dosage schedule or every form of application used is entirely at the user's own risk and responsibility.** The authors and publishers request every user to report to the publishers any discrepancies or inaccuracies noticed.

Preface

Perfusion is defined as the steady state delivery of blood to tissue. Many physiologists use the term "perfusion" to emphasize contact with the tissue, or in other words *capillary* blood flow. Because blood flow brings crucial nutrients, and because it is disturbed in many disease processes, monitoring of this key physiological parameter can often provide insight into disease. Consequently, the measurement of perfusion for medical purposes has been performed in almost all organs using many techniques. Rather than survey the entire field of perfusion imaging, this book focuses on the use of MRI and, in particular, MRI combined with contrast agents to assess hemodynamics in only one organ: the brain. While MRI has traditionally been used to evaluate anatomy, with its main application being the CNS, the recent application of MRI to visualize tissue physiology or function has met with great success. Indeed, a whole new field known as functional MRI has arisen to apply these techniques. Because blood flow is altered in many pathophysiological states, from abnormal cognition through stroke to brain tumors, use of MRI to study blood flow is one of the most clinically relevant of the many forms of functional MRI.

Over the past 10 years, considerable experience has been accrued using contrast agents to measure cerebral hemodynamics with MRI [1, 2, 2a, 2b]. The basic technique is to inject a gadolinium chelate and acquire images rapidly as the bolus of contrast agent passes through the blood vessels in the brain [3]. The contrast agent causes a signal change; this signal change over time can then be analyzed to measure cerebral hemodynamics. The ability to perform perfusion MRI is now becoming widespread as the necessary hardware and software become increasingly available. Because so many diseases of the brain can be better diagnosed and perhaps even better managed by assessing brain hemodynamics, the demand for information about how to perform and interpret these techniques has grown substantially. Fortunately, perfusion MRI can be performed with nearly all up-to-date clinical scanners using a combination of rapid imaging techniques and the bolus injection of clinically approved extracellular gadolinium chelates. The details of how to do this, however, remain incompletely understood to many; hence the rationale for this book.

This book will familiarize the reader with the basic principles of perfusion MR imaging. All relevant technical aspects are addressed (we hope!), contrast agents are described, imaging protocols are provided, and the postprocessing of images is described. Dedicated software for personal use of the reader for postprocessing of images and further analysis is provided on a disc. In addition to the technical details of acquisition and post processing, numerous examples of the application of these tools in the clinical setting are also described. In particular, the book includes a discussion of the role of perfusion MRI in the current evaluation of cerebrovascular disease, including an integrative approach using diffusion MR imaging in conjunction with perfusion imaging. We will also discuss the role of perfusion MRI in the assessment of cerebral neoplasia, and discuss some of the challenges and opportunities that imaging tumors present. Some of the particular strengths of perfusion MRI, such as its relatively high resolution and possible microvascular specificity, will be discussed. The book includes an extensive bibliography.

If you are completely new to perfusion MRI, then we might suggest that you read Part 2: Perfusion Imaging in Clinical Practice, before Part 1: Technical Considerations. Many of the technical details about perfusion MRI become relevant only once an understanding of perfusion MRI's capabilities are clear. Once you understand what perfusion MRI is capable of, then read Part 1 to understand how to acquire and post-process the images. Then, with that knowledge, reread Part 2 to understand some of the subtleties that are best appreciated when both the technical and clinical information can be appreciated.

Charlestown, early 2000   A. Gregory Sorensen
Karlsruhe   Peter Reimer

Acknowledgements

We wish to thank most of all the pioneering leadership of the "prime mover" of perfusion MRI, Bruce Rosen. Without his scientific vision and (in both of our cases) his direct teaching and training, this book would not have been possible. We feel fortunate to count him as a trusted friend and mentor. We also wish to thank the series of researchers whose hard work, foresight, and intellectual horsepower has brought perfusion MRI into the clinical realm. While there is not room to list all of the people who have contributed to this effort over the years, a short list must include: Hannu Aronen, Jack Belliveau, Thomas Brady, Jerry Boxerman, William Copen, Timothy Davis, Ken Kwong, Michael Lev, Robert McKinstry, Leif Østergaard, Arno Villringer, Robert Weisskoff, and Ona Wu. Additional thanks goes to those who have helped with figures, contributed patient information, or provided other assistance. This includes Jerome Beers, Gilberto Gonzalez, Griffith Harsh, Frank Pardo, Megan Salhus, Pamela Schaefer, Verdene Smith, Jennifer Synnott, Andrew Tievsky, Alan Thornton, Mike Vevea, Larry Wald, Kei Yamada, Takashi Yoshiura, and Greg Zaharchuk.

Table of Contents

List of Abbreviations

ASL	Arterial Spin Labeling
BBB	Blood-Brain Barrier
CBF	Cerebral Blood Flow
CBV	Cerebral Blood Volume
CNS	Central Nervous System
CT	Computed Tomography
EPI	Echo Planar Imaging
FLASH	Fast Low Angle Shot
Gd	Gadolinium
GE	Gradient Echo
ICA	Internal Carotid Artery
MCA	Middle Cerebral Artery
MRA	Magnetic Resonance Angiography
MRI	Magnetic Resonance Imaging
MTT	Mean Transit Time
PET	Positron Emission Tomography
ROI	Region of Interest
SE	Spin Echo
SNR	Signal to Noise Ratio
SPECT	Single Photon Emission Computed Tomography
SPIO	Superparamagnetic Iron Oxides
TE	Echo time
TR	Repetition time
VEGF	Vascular Endothelial Growth Factor

List of Movie Clips

Part 1: Technical Considerations

Introduction

In performing perfusion MRI, or indeed any functional MRI technique, an important concept to keep in mind is that of compromise. There are many variables to optimize with perfusion MRI – pulse sequence use, TR, TE, type of injection, spatial resolution, etc. Implementing perfusion MRI in your own clinical or research practice will likely mean making trade-offs between these. For example, if one chooses a very short TR, then the number of slices may be decreased compared to a longer TR. However, this need for compromise is actually good news; it means that there are usually many ways to acquire data, and that there is flexibility in looking for solutions. As we describe our own opinions on the best way to solve some of the technical challenges of perfusion MRI, remember that our recommendations might shift if and when higher performance systems become available, or if a new contrast agent is introduced. The goal of this book is to provide the reader with enough information to be able to perform her or his own optimization for the equipment, personnel, and needs at hand. While we will offer specific recommendations frequently, we will try to explain the reasons for these recommendations so that they can be adapted to each local situation appropriately.

Cerebral hemodynamics – what are they?

Before we begin to describe how to measure cerebral hemodynamics, it is useful to describe what exactly it is that we are measuring. Perfusion is the steady state delivery of blood to tissue parenchyma through the capillaries, representing the microscopic coherent motion of water and cellular material. Perfusion is typically measured in mL/100 g of tissue/min, or units of CBF. Normal human gray matter is perfused at a rate of 50 – 60 mL/100 g/min and is maintained in a narrow range by cerebral autoregulation. Thus, low perfusion states might result in cellular ischemia, and high perfusion states might be associated with hypervascular lesions such as some tumors.

Fig. 1 A shows a simple pipe. By inserting a known amount of a tracer, such as a dye, into the pipe, and then watching to see when it comes out, we can learn something about the pipe and the flow through it. In particular, when the dye exits will depend on how big the pipe is (the volume of the pipe) and how fast the flow is. In simple terms the flow multiplied by the circulation time, or the time the dye takes to get through the pipe, equals the volume of the pipe. The units for this make sense: flow is in mL/min; circulation time is in min, and multiplying those units together yields mL, or a volume measurement. Hence, measuring flow can be done if the volume and circulation or transit time is known.

As we consider the application of the simple illustration above to the brain, we realize that in addition to CBF, cerebral hemodynamics encompass other parameters. One particularly relevant parameter is cerebral blood volume. CBV differs from CBF in that CBV is the amount of blood in a given amount of tissue at any time – the size of the pipe,

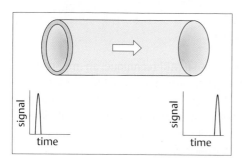

Fig. 1   Diagrams of measurement of a tracer (signal) versus time at various points in an idealized pipe.

(**A**) Simple schema of blood flow through a pipe. Tracer is injected into the pipe at a known rate as shown in the graph on the left. If the flow in the pipe is constant the tracer will be detected exiting the pipe at the same rate as it was injected as illustrated in the graph on the right.

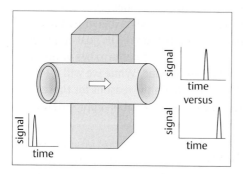

(**B**) If the injection occurs at a known time as shown on the graph on the left, but the rate of flow through the pipe is not known, one can determine the flow rate based on the time that the injection is detected. If it is early, as in the upper right graph, then the flow is faster than if it arrives later, as depicted in the graph on the lower right. Indeed the flow rate and the volume of the pipe can both be determined from the concentration of the agent over time in this simple example.

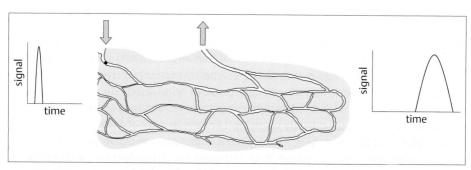

(**C**) When the pipe is not single but a network of varying sized pipes, such as a capillary bed, then the simple approaches above are no longer valid. Broadening of the output measurement could be due to slow flow in any one of the segments. Determining flow becomes even more complicated if the injection of the tracer is not done in a known manner.

so to speak – while CBF represents the amount of blood *moving through* a given amount of tissue per unit time. The simple relationship of

flow × circulation time = volume

helps relate these in both an idealized and a clinical setting.

Changes in CBF and CBV are typically well correlated, meaning that when CBV rises, so does CBF, and vice versa [4]. To continue along with the pipe analogy, one might imagine that larger pipes often have faster flow through them. However, CBV and CBF become uncorrelated in some pathological states. For example, in acute cerebral ischemia, the vascular bed may dilate in a compensatory response to decreased perfusion pressure, and thus raise CBV. This is due to a lack of flow (that is, low CBF); this mismatch between CBV and CBF can be quite dramatic and is a familiar finding in acute ischemic stroke [5–8]. Blood volume is an important parameter because it is so simple to measure: the amount of signal change is proportional to the concentration of the tracer. Indeed, it is often the relative concentration of an agent at a given point of time that is easiest to measure. This is the case with MRI as well as with X-ray computed tomography. In the case of MRI, however, the relaxation rate affects the signal with an exponential relationship rather than a linear relationship, and with a drop in signal at high concentrations rather than an increase in signal. Specifically, it is the log of the signal drop in a voxel after administration of the agent that is (roughly) proportional to the amount of contrast in the voxel. This relationship means that CBV is a robust, reliable parameter; indeed, it can be determined even if first pass imaging cannot be obtained.

Another hemodynamic parameter is the mean transit time of the tracer through the tissue. MTT is strictly defined as CBV divided by CBF, and hence it corresponds to the "circulation time" mentioned above. Unfortunately, the colloquial use of the term "MTT" is inappropriately much broader such that MTT is often incorrectly used to refer to the duration of the signal change in a voxel on dynamic MRI, which is not the same thing as the circulation time [9]. Many timing parameters are used as indicators of cerebral hemodynamics, chiefly because they are easy to compute. These are discussed in detail below; the most popular include the time to the peak signal change after the bolus was injected (termed "time to peak"), and the time of arrival of the bolus in a voxel ("arrival time"). Another popular parameter is the width of the curve representing the signal drop over time; the width is usually measured at half the height of the curve, so-called "full width half maximum" or FWHM. Each one of these various metrics – CBV, CBF, time to peak, MTT, etc., – is an attempt to gauge what is happening to the tracer, and therefore to the vascular bed. Fortunately, each of these parameters can be computed on a voxel-by-voxel basis, and displayed as an image. Fig. 2 demonstrates examples of these parameter maps. (Incidentally, note the difference in flow and volume in the gray matter versus the white matter. This normal difference can often obscure subtle changes and has raised interest in images like the MTT images that have a uniform appearance in normal areas.)

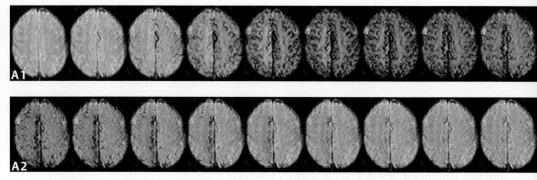

Fig. **2** Sample raw data and parameter maps from a patient suffering from acute stroke symptoms. A 64-year-old woman was imaged 5.5 hours after the onset of left-sided weakness.

(**A**) Sequential gradient echo, echo-planar images (GE EPI, TR = 1,5 s) demonstrating transient signal drop as the contrast agent passes through the brain. Note the transient signal drop and the subsequent return. Compare these still images to Movie Clip ⊙ **1**, a normal perfusion study, and Movie Clip ⊙ **2**, this same patient's study in cine mode.

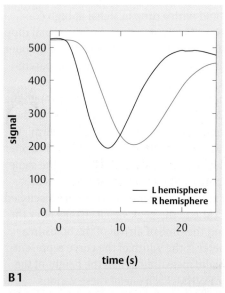

B 1

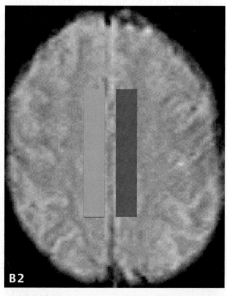

B 2

(**B**) Graph of signal versus time for two regions of interest in the left and right hemisphere. Note the delay in the peak signal drop in the right hemisphere compared to the left. This delay can be imaged using a variety of parametric maps, shown in the following images. Each of these maps consists of a parameter computed at each voxel, and a new map synthesized of such values.

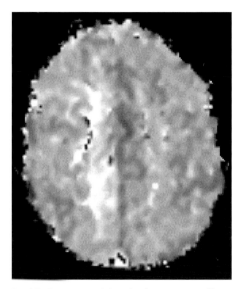

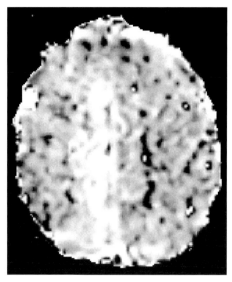

2 (**C**) Time to peak (TTP). This is a map of how long from the injection of the contrast agent (or the start of imaging) to the time of peak signal drop. This is a relatively straightforward and computationally simple metric to compute.

2 (**D**) The width of the signal change curve at half of its maximum change, known as full width at half maximum (FWHM).

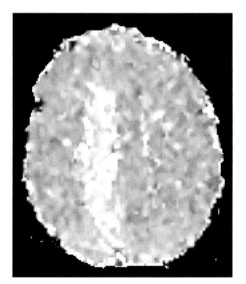

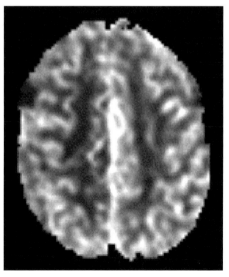

2 (**E**) Arrival time. This is calculated by estimating when the signal begins to drop. It typically is less well defined than the peak signal change or FWHM because of noise around the baseline.

2 (**F**) Relative CBF, computed using the method described in [2a].

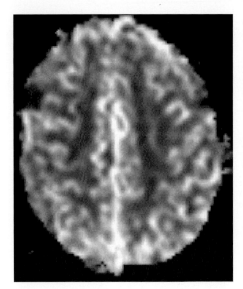

2   (**G**) Relative CBV.

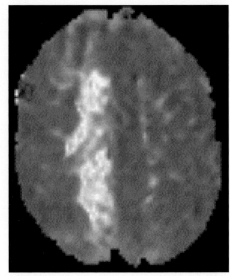

2   (**H**) MTT, calculated as CBV divided by CBF (on a voxel-by-voxel basis). Note that the timing maps demonstrate an obvious abnormality, while the same area on the CBV and CBF maps appears more normal. This is probably due to threshold effects: even small timing changes can appear significant.

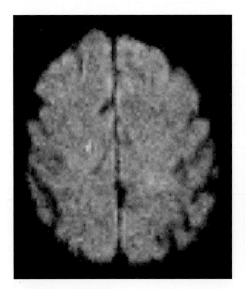

2   (**I**) The initial DWI.

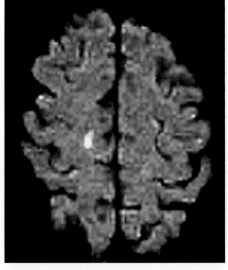

2   (**J**) 2 day follow-up DWI. Note that initial and follow-up DWI demonstrate that a much smaller area has proceeded to infarction than the timing maps might predict. The CBF and CBV maps, however, appear to be more accurate. Reasons for this are discussed in part 2 of this book.

Table **1** Values for common perfusion parameters in normal adult humans

Parameter	Value in gray matter (white matter values are about half that of gray matter)
CBF	About 50 mL/100 g/min
CBV	About 4 mL/100 mL of tissue
MTT [$\equiv$ CBV/CBF]	About 5 seconds

Importantly, there is a clear distinction between studying the tissue of interest with perfusion imaging and studying it with MRA. While both detect blood flow, they focus on different flows in different vessels. MRA has demonstrated its ability to detect flow in macroscopic vasculature (arteries and veins, primarily) and is widely used to detect arterial or venous disease. However, much of CNS pathology begins at the cellular and tissue level and is not accompanied by any alteration of the macroscopic circulation; instead, the capillaries, arterioles, or venules are where the pathophysiological changes occur. As a result, MRA can be insensitive to many pathologies, particularly in their early stages. Perfusion imaging, on the other hand, is concerned with microscopic flow; that is, flow at the capillary level, and therefore can potentially detect such changes at an early stage. Table **1** lists some common values for CBF, CBV, and their quotient, MTT.

Tissue perfusion has been assessed using a variety of radiological techniques, from conventional catheter angiography to PET and SPECT. While a detailed analysis of each of these competing techniques is beyond the scope of this primer, MRI does have unique features that add to its value in assessing tissue perfusion in the brain. For example, MRI can be relatively sensitive to tissue microvasculature, it is minimally invasive, and has higher spatial resolution than radionuclide-based techniques, and better contrast-to-noise per unit time compared to X-ray computed tomography. Its lack of radiation also gives it a somewhat improved safety profile compared to CT perfusion, and the ability of MRI to collect rapidly repeated images at multiple slices is unmatched by even the newest CT technologies.

Perfusion MRI with dynamic susceptibility contrast imaging

The most popular way of performing perfusion MRI is to inject a contrast agent and observe its passage through the brain [10–13]. Table **2** lists some common parameters for performing a routine perfusion study in the brain. First described in the brain by Villringer et al. [3], contrast-based hemodynamic perfusion imaging with MRI has been applied to a variety of clinical applications including tumor characterization, stroke, and dementia, with others under active investigation. With currently available MR contrast media (gadolinium chelates), the physical basis of these techniques rests on dynamic imaging during the first passage of a contrast agent bolus. MRI users are familiar with Gd chelates, as they typically cause signal enhancement. However, the short range, dipole-dipole (relaxivity) effects conventionally used to affect T1 contrast depend upon a contrast agent's direct access to water molecules to perturb the MR signal. In the brain, this access is effectively limited to the intravascular space in the presence of an intact blood-brain barrier (BBB). In normal brain tissue, therefore, there is little or no enhancement. Rather than using T1 effects, the Gd chelate is used as a tracer by virtue of its T2 and T2* effects. This is because on the first pass through the brain vessels, a rapidly injected bolus of contrast media maintains a high enough concentration such that the T2 effects outweigh the T1 effects. These T2 relaxation effects are highlighted by the compartmentalization of the agent in the vessels. This com-

Table **2**   Common parameters for perfusion MRI of the brain

Parameter	Typical Value
TR	1500 ms
TE	70 ms
FOV	20 cm × 20 cm
Matrix	128 × 128
Slice thickness	5 or 6 mm
Interslice gap	1 mm or interleaved
Number of repeated images at each slice	45
Number of slices	11
Total imaging time	TR × number of repeated images = 45 × 1.5 = 68 seconds
Time of injection	10 seconds after imaging begins
Amount of contrast	0.2 mmol/kg (e.g., 40 mL for a 100 kg person)
Rate of injection	5 mL/second
Amount of saline flush	25 mL
Rate of saline flush	5 mL/second
Size of iv catheter	18 gauge or larger (although as small as 22 gauge can be used if necessary)

These parameters have been used extensively at 1.5 T, on a General Electric Signa MRI system modified for EPI by Advanced NMR Systems. Similar protocols are applicable to other systems; see Table **4** for further discussion.

partmentalization means that the magnetic field induced by the susceptibility of the contrast agent is different inside the vessels than outside; this in turn leads to T2 and T2* relaxation resulting in signal loss [14–16].

The basis of magnetic susceptibility (T2 and/or T2*) contrast results from microscopic variations in the magnetic field that are caused by the heterogeneous distribution of high magnetic susceptibility contrast agents within a tissue. This microscopic heterogeneity of magnetic field leads to a loss of transverse phase coherence and hence to a loss of MRI signal. This mechanism is identical to that invoked to explain the loss of signal during hemorrhagic disease characterized by compartmentalization of iron, as either deoxygenated intact red cells acutely or as ferritin/hemosiderin clumps chronically. Image contrast in susceptibility-contrast (T2 or T2*) studies is occasioned by longer range (in the order of microns) rather than molecular (in the order of ångstroms) magnetic field perturbations that the paramagnetic agents produce when compartmentalized within the vascular bed. Within this space, these magnetic susceptibility effects relax the transverse magnetization of *surrounding* tissue protons for a distance roughly equal to the radius of the blood vessel. Fig. **3** demonstrates how at low concentration there is minimal effect on spins outside the vessel but at high concentration, the effects extend beyond the capillary and into the surrounding tissues.

Since this magnetic susceptibility contrast phenomenon is due to the high concentration of Gd, it is diminished after the first pass of the agent through the brain due to dilution of the agent. Therefore, rapid imaging is required to measure the first pass tissue transit of intravenously administered contrast materials. Such data can then be analyzed using the same tracer kinetic principles developed for other tracers to measure cerebral blood flow and volume. To use these approaches to determine relative CBV or CBF, it is necessary to convert changes in MR signal intensity with respect to time into contrast agent tissue concentration-versus-time curves. Both theoretical and empirical studies have shown that the degree of signal drop in a voxel depends on the amount of agent in a voxel [12,17]. This in turn relies on two factors: the concentration of an injected contrast agent within the blood and the fractional volume of intravascular space within the tissue (the cerebral blood volume). This relationship between the measured signal change over time and the concentration of tracer in a voxel over time is the key link that allows measurement of cerebral hemodynamics.

This use of signal change to calculate cerebral hemodynamics need not be complex. For example, since there is a relationship between the amount of signal change in a voxel and the amount of contrast agent in the voxel, one might simply compare precontrast to post-contrast images; the change in signal should be only due to the addition of the contrast agent (and noise). This signal change can be related to concentration; the concentration can then be used to estimate blood volume. The SNR of this measurement can be improved by repeatedly measuring the change, and then integrating (or summing) the signal change over time; that is, acquiring multiple images before and multiple images after the injection of the agent and comparing the average "before" image with the average "after" image. Fig. **4** shows a graph of signal versus

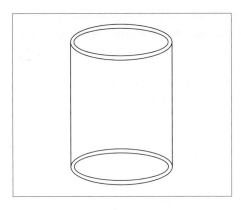

Fig. 3   Basic mechanism of susceptibility physics.

(**A**) The magnetic field inside a tube such as a capillary and outside are relatively similar. Therefore, as spins (water) move in and around the capillary, no significant dephasing occurs.

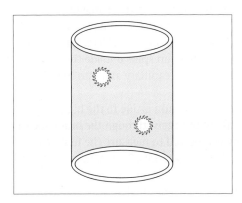

(**B**) At low concentration, such as five minutes after injection of a standard dose, only a few gadolinium-containing molecules are in each tube. This allows T1 relaxation of those spins (water molecules) that approach the Gd molecules closely. However, the overall magnetic field is not changed much in the capillary.

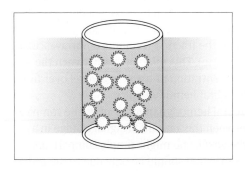

(**C**) At high concentration, such as during the first pass of a bolus injection, there are enough Gd molecules to change the magnetic field within the capillary as compared to that outside the capillaries. This is because the magnetic susceptibility of the inside of the capillary with the paramagnetic contrast agent is different than the diamagnetic tissue outside the capillary. This means that there is a difference in magnetic field, or a gradient, between the region inside the capillary and the outside. As spins move from inside the capillary to outside, they see a changing magnetic field; this in turns causes T2 and T2* relaxation. This increased relaxation leads to signal loss in the voxel.

time during the injection of a contrast agent, and the conversion of this to a graph of delta R2, which is linearly related to concentration. This approach of measuring concentration of an MRI-visible tracer over time is similar to tracer experiments used in nuclear medicine. Unlike conventional nuclear medicine studies, however, the degree of signal change that results from the susceptibility effect of a given injection of contrast is highly dependent on the specific acquisition technique used.

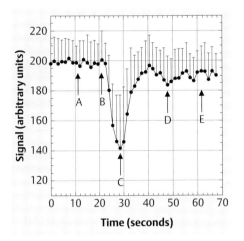 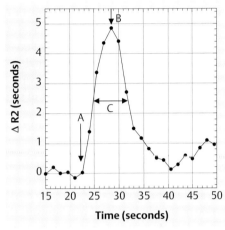

Fig. 4 Normal signal vs. time graph and R2 vs. time graph. These graphs were made from data obtained by placing a region of interest over an area of gray matter in a normal subject (the same subject as in Movie Clip ⊙ **1**).

(A) Graph of normal signal versus time curve. Arrows highlight various recognizable components of the curve. Error bars represent the standard deviation in the ROI.

A: Baseline region. These images establish what the signal is before the contrast arrives.

B: Arrival point of contrast agent. If there are few baseline data or if the baseline is highly variable, determining the true arrival time can be difficult.

C: Peak signal change. This corresponds to when the highest concentration of contrast agent is present. After this peak there is reduced contrast agent as the bolus washes out of the brain, and therefore the signal begins to normalize.

D: A second small peak in the signal drop is identified due to recirculation of the bolus.

E: Note that the post-injection signal intensity is slightly lower than the pre-injection baseline. This is because during the first few minutes, the concentration of Gd is still high enough that there is a slight susceptibility difference between the intravascular and extravascular spaces, leading to a small amount of signal loss.

(B) A graph of a portion of the data on the left, converted to change in R2 (the inverse of T2) versus time. Again one can see A, the arrival time, and B, the peak signal change. Because high R2 means a much shorter T2 and therefore a bigger signal loss, the curve is inverted compared to the graph on the left. However, it is also more analogous to the concentration of Gd at a given point. Point C is the width at half-maximum, so called FWHM. At about 48 seconds the recirculation peak can again be noted. Blood volume can be calculated from the area of this ΔR2 curve, and if the arterial input function is known, blood flow information can also be extracted.

Why is magnetic susceptibility so powerful?

Gadolinium agents have two effects: they shorten T1, causing signal enhancement on T1-weighted images, and at high concentration also shorten T2, causing signal decrease on T2-weighted images [12]. While the T1 effects take place at short range – that is, the spins to be shortened must be very close to the Gd atom – the T2 effects can take place over a longer range [14,15]. Hence, the key reason that susceptibility contrast is so effective is because the susceptibility effect extends *outside* the capillaries. Only 4% of the volume of a voxel of gray matter is inside the capillaries (and even less in white matter). This means that if we had to depend on the intravascular effects of our agent alone, then we would only change the signal in 4% of the spins. However, the susceptibility effect lets more spins be affected – potentially *all* of the spins in a voxel. By affecting more spins, we get a bigger change in signal with a susceptibility effect than with an intravascular-only effect. This improved signal means better images.

Why use contrast agents?

The susceptibility effect can actually be detected without extrinsic contrast agents; this is one of the fundamental mechanisms that is felt to underlie the blood oxygen level dependent (BOLD) techniques used for activation mapping in the brain [18–20]. In this case, the contrast agent is an intrinsic one: hemoglobin. As it changes oxygenation state, its susceptibility effects change [21]. However, these changes are minor – in the order of 1% at 1.5 Tesla, and difficult to produce uniformly throughout the brain. On the other hand, with the injection of gadolinium-based agents there can be signal change of 20% or more, depending on the dose of contrast agent and imaging pulse sequence used [1,3,11]. Hence, the rationale for using contrast agents is to simply take advantage of their larger susceptibility effect, and thereby improve visualization of blood flow, blood volume, and brain function. In short, the passage of an exogenous contrast agent like Gd induces a more significant change in signal than intrinsic markers like hemoglobin or spin-tagging techniques (at least using currently available techniques). Since creating meaningful images of cerebral hemodynamics is so dependent on good signal-to-noise ratios, the improvement in SNR offered by contrast agents is a key factor in their popularity for perfusion MRI.

Exogenous contrast agents well suited for demonstrating perfusion include paramagnetic agents (gadolinium and dysprosium), macromolecular agents (e.g., gadolinium bound to albumin or other macromolecules), superparamagnetic nanoparticles (e.g., iron oxide particles), or microbubbles. Clinically available gadolinium chelates have a much stronger susceptibility effect than deoxyhemoglobin (which is also paramagnetic as indicated above). At present, no macromolecular agents or microbubbles are approved clinically for MRI, although clinical trials are underway. A formulation of iron oxide particles is available (ferumoxides injectable solution), although not approved for bolus use.

Bolus injection versus slow infusion of contrast agent

There are two reasons why a bolus injection of Gd-based agent is important for cerebral perfusion imaging. First of all, it is only in their concentrated form that Gd-based agents have significant T2 effects. At low concentrations, the T1 effects dominate; to achieve a high concentration in the brain the contrast agent must remain relatively concentrated. Because the current generation of Gd agents are extracellular agents and freely pass out of the vasculature in the body, the concentration of Gd is too small to cause a significant signal change if the Gd is not injected as a bolus. Indeed, other studies of the chelating molecules (such as DTPA) suggest that approximately 20% of the DTPA passes into the extravascular space on the first pass through the lungs alone. Infusing as a slow drip would preclude any T2 effects and therefore prevent any significant measurement of cerebral hemodynamics.

The second reason is related to the measurement of blood flow, rather than only blood volume. Blood volume actually can be measured using steady-state techniques, and in fact steady-state measurements of blood volume have been done with use of T2 agents and MRI [22]. However, while the steady-state approach can measure blood volume well, it cannot measure blood flow well. The very nature of steady state imaging is to ignore flow information; it is concerned with whether or not contrast agent has arrived, not how fast it arrived or how fast it is leaving. Of course, blood flow is an important component of cerebral hemodynamics, so techniques to measure it are of interest. This requires a bolus approach, and the more narrow the bolus the better the measurement of flow can be. Ideally, when using exogenous contrast agents one would prefer an infinitely narrow bolus of contrast (what mathematicians term a "delta function"). However, the ideal is never realized because of the trade-offs involved. For example, the bolus of contrast could be narrower if an intra-arterial injection were performed. However, this is not realistic in routine practice, and so instead we decide to trade off the precision that would come from such invasive approaches for a less precise but more clinically feasible approach. Nonetheless, a narrow bolus is still preferable (as it is even for CBV imaging [23]); methods to narrow the bolus width include more rapid intravenous injections (such as are obtainable with a power injector) and/or a more concentrated agent (such as a dysprosium-based agent or a more highly concentrated gadolinium agent). Note that such improvements should improve maps of CBF, but not necessarily those of CBV, since CBV can be measured with a steady-state approach. Fig. **5** illustrates a typical MR-compatible power injector.

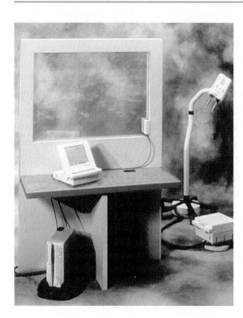

Fig. 5   A typical MR-compatible power injector (photo courtesy of Medrad Inc.).

Why is the status of the BBB important for Perfusion MRI?

At the time of writing (early 2000), clinically available gadolinium chelates are extracellular low-molecular weight molecules (550–600 Daltons) which are not specific for the vascular space and instead equilibrate across the interstitial space. For first-pass perfusion studies in the brain, however, the effects of interstitial equilibration are much less marked than they would be in other tissues, since the BBB holds the extracellular low-molecular paramagnetic chelates within the vascular space. Therefore, in the presence of an intact or only minimally disrupted BBB the current class of extracellular gadolinium chelates effectively become intravascular agents in the CNS. Since the contrast agent is intravascular, it can produce only T1 shortening (and thereby signal enhancement) of the blood pool itself. Of course, the intravascular agent can produce T2 shortening – and the susceptibility effects we depend on for perfusion MRI – inside and outside the vessels. Following disruption of the blood-brain barrier, low-molecular gadolinium chelates equilibrate across the BBB, entering both the intravascular and the extravascular compartments. This produces two effects that counteract the susceptibility contrast mechanism: first, there is a decrease in compartmentalization; as described above compartmentalization is the crucial component required for susceptibility imaging. Second, even a small amount of extravascular Gd causes T1 shortening of the tissue outside the intravascular space and hence a signal increase in the 96% of tissue that is not within the vessels. This signal increase can counteract the signal decrease expected from the susceptibility effect. Because of these two synergistic mechanisms, even a mildly leaky BBB can lead to a lack of susceptibility effect. What effect might this have on perfusion MRI? In the worst case, this leakiness can lead to what appears to be absent or even "negative" blood volume, since the signal increase from T1 effects can counterbalance the signal decrease from T2 effects. Fig. **6** demonstrates how a leaky BBB can affect the CBV calculation.

Of course, like many things in MRI, what is a disadvantage in one setting can, with some clever work, be turned into an advantage. For some moderate degrees of BBB breakdown, algorithms to compensate for this effect have been created (e.g., by Weisskoff et al. [24]). These correction algorithms in fact allow not only the compensation of CBV maps for breakdown of the BBB, but also provide an estimate of permeability. (Formally speaking, they provide an estimate of the permeability multiplied by the surface area of the vascular bed in a given voxel.) A number of approaches to measuring BBB permeability with MRI have been proposed; the elegance of the Weisskoff technique is that the permeability data are acquired simultaneously with perfusion MRI data.

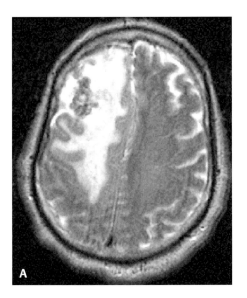

Fig. **6**   Effect of blood-brain barrier on computation of cerebral blood volume.

(**A**) T2-weighted image showing focal metastasis surrounded by edema in the right frontal lobe of a 65-year-old male.

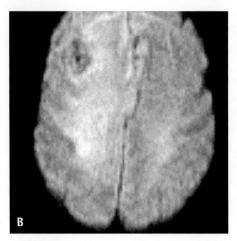

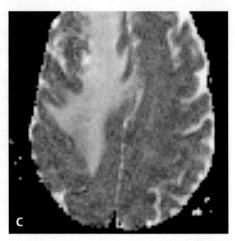

6 (**B**) Diffusion-weighted image and (**C**) map of apparent diffusion coefficient confirm the vasogenic edema surrounding the lesion.

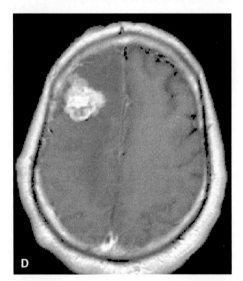

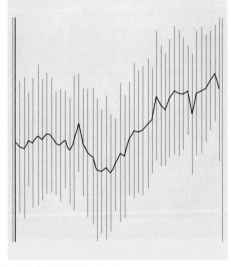

6 (**D**) Marked enhancement after the administration of Gd is noted.

6 (**E**) The signal versus time curve for a region of interest in the lesion demonstrates that the signal first drops and then rises, indicating competing T1 and T2 effects. (The dark line is the mean signal intensity in the ROI, the blue lines represent the standard deviation in the ROI.)

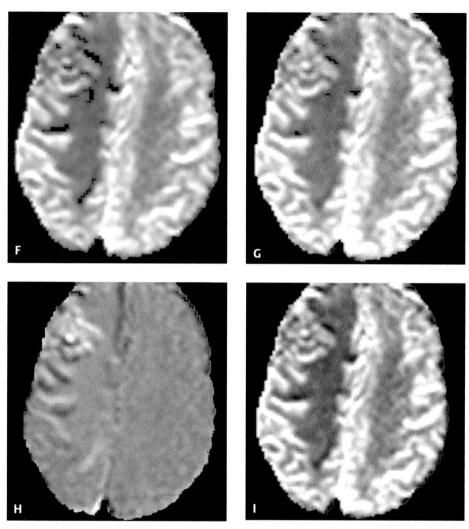

6   (**F**) Uncorrected CBV maps suggest that much of the lesion has lower CBV than gray matter. This seems unlikely given the highly angiogenic nature of metastasis.

Correction maps including estimates of blood volume (**G**) and permeability-surface area product (**H**) demonstrate that there is substantial leakage present; incorporating these together allows computation of a corrected CBV map (**I**) that demonstrates high CBV in the lesion. See also Movie Clip ⊙ **3**.

How do I image perfusion in the presence of a leaky BBB?

There are at least two options available to help perfusion MRI in the presence of a leaky BBB, and we recommend using both of them if possible. First, one can "pre-dose" with 0.025 or 0.05 mmol/kg of Gd five to ten minutes before the bolus injection, then use the remaining 0.15 to 0.2 mmol/kg for the main injection. The benefits of this accrue by allowing the extravascular space to have its T1 shortened by the pre-dose of Gd. In the presence of a very leaky BBB, even the small dose of Gd that constitutes the pre-dose will allow substantial T1 shortening to occur, because even a small amount of Gd can cause relaxation quite efficiently. Then, when the main bolus of Gd arrives, there is no more relaxation to be done. In effect, the enhancement has already occurred, so there is no longer competition between T2 shortening (leading to signal drop) and T1 shortening (leading to signal increase). While this does not overcome the decreased signal drop due to decreased compartmentalization, there is still a substantial benefit in our experience. Since this costs little in the instances where there is no BBB (breakdown), a standardized protocol can be used where the pre-dose is given during, say, the T2 axial imaging (but after the FLAIR imaging).

The other option available is to use a postprocessing approach to try and compensate for the BBB breakdown, such as the Weisskoff technique described above. We typically use both approaches to minimize BBB breakdown side effects. In the future, an agent with less T1 effects, such as an iron oxide agent or a dysprosium-based agent, may also help with this problem.

Advantages of available and future contrast agents

Currently, several extracellular gadolinium chelates are clinically approved and are all supplied at a 0.5 molar concentration (Table **3**). Gadolinium (Gd) belongs to the class of lanthanide (rare earth) metals and possesses a large magnetic moment because of seven unpaired $4f$ suborbital electrons. Gadolinium-based contrast agents are clinically used to enhance the signal intensity of tissue on T1-weighted images. Gadolinium is chelated with low molecular-weight ligands and the complexes are quite similar from a pharmacological point of view. They have similar excretion and equilibration constants. As mentioned above they each remain in the intravascular space of the CNS if the BBB is intact, and they accumulate in the interstitial space if there is no barrier as in other organs or if the BBB is not intact. None of these agents are blood pool agents, because they are not limited to the intravascular space, nor are they tissue specific. Nevertheless, they are of course widely used. These agents include gadopentetate dimeglumine, gadodiamide, gadoteridol, and gadolinium-DO3 A. All approved agents can be injected at a dose of 0.1 mmol gadolinium/kg body weight; some are also approved for administration of 0.3 mmol gadolinium/kg body weight. While no agent is currently approved for the specific indication of cerebral perfusion imaging, each

Table **3**   Approved gadolinium chelates useful for perfusion imaging (listed in order of regulatory approval)

Contrast agents	Trade name	Company
0.5 molar		
Gadopentetate dimeglumine	Magnevist	Schering & Berlex
Gadodiamide	Omniscan	Nycomed-Amersham
Gadoteridol	ProHance	Bracco
Gadolinium-DO3 A	Dotarem	Guerbet
Gadobenate dimeglumine	MultiHance	Bracco
Gadoversetamide	OptiMARK	Mallinckrodt
1.0 molar		
Gadobutrol	Gadovist	Schering

Gd-based agent can be useful for this purpose, and such usage is in conformance with the agents' approved role as an aid to diagnosis of intracranial pathology.

More recently, a higher concentrated gadolinium chelate has been developed and clinically evaluated, and has been approved for use in some countries. This new neutral gadolinium chelate "gadobutrol", (Gadovist; Schering AG, Berlin) is provided as a 1.0 molar formulation. This higher concentration allows one to proportionally decrease the injection volume. This in turn makes the bolus narrower. Therefore, this agent appears to be particularly well-suited for perfusion (blood flow) imaging because the susceptibility effects are more pronounced as a result of the compactness of the bolus. Figs. **7 A, B** demonstrate signal changes as a function of dose in a group of normal volunteers.

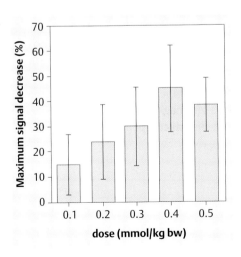

Fig. **7**   (**A**) Perfusion imaging with concentrated agents.

Maximum decrease in cortical signal intensity during perfusion imaging with gadobutrol using T2*-weighted FLASH with an injection rate of 5 ml/s is shown. Studies were performed in 80 subjects assessing five different doses. The dose of 0.3 mmol/kg gadobutrol was considered to be sufficient for clinical perfusion imaging.

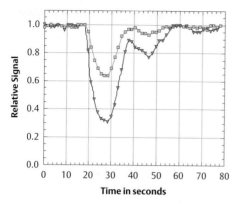 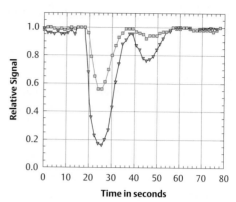

7 **(B)** Shown above are data comparing 0.3 mmol/kg gadopentate dimeglumine (left) with 0.3 mmol/kg gadobutrol (right). Open squares represent the signal in a ROI placed in gray matter, whereas the triangles represent the signal in a ROI placed near the MCA, the same as an AIF. The peak signal drop is greater and also narrower with gadobutrol due to its increased concentration for the same overall dose. See also Movie Clips ⊙ **4** and **5**.

Dysprosium-based agents are another class of contrast agents that would be favorable for perfusion imaging. Dysprosium (Dy) is also a lanthanide metal and closely related to gadolinium with similar physical and chemical characteristics. Theoretically, dysprosium is better suited for susceptibility-contrast perfusion imaging compared with gadolinium because of a 1.8 times stronger susceptibility effect and a weaker T1 relaxivity effect as compared to gadolinium chelates (the T1 relaxivity of Dy is about 2.5% that of Gd). A compound chelated with DTPA-BMA (dysprosium-DTPA-BMA, sprodiamide; Nycomed) was studied with doses from 0.1 – 0.3 mmol dysprosium/kg body weight in humans. The enhancement caused by dysprosium appeared to be twice as great as that of gadolinium, being consistent with the higher magnetic susceptibility of dysprosium. To the extent that they behave similarly to gadolinium chelates, dysprosium chelates are sensitive to the same inaccuracies as gadolinium chelates in the presence of a damaged BBB. That is, there will be loss of compartmentalization resulting in diminished T2 effects in areas of severe BBB breakdown. While there might be diminished T2 effects, there are few T1 effects to compete with the T2 effects, which should be an advantage for Dy-based compounds for imaging perfusion in the presence of BBB breakdown. It remains unclear whether a clinical compound will become available.

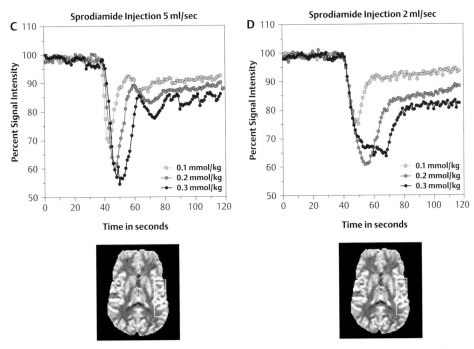

7 (**C**) Injection of sprodiamide (Dy-DTPA-BMA) at 5 mL/s, and (**D**) at 2 mL/s. Note how the slower injection rate allows blurring together of the first and second passes of the bolus at the highest dose.

Figs. **7 C, D** demonstrate the superior imaging characteristics of this compound, and Fig. **8** shows sample images of perfusion studies done with Dy-DTPA-BMA.

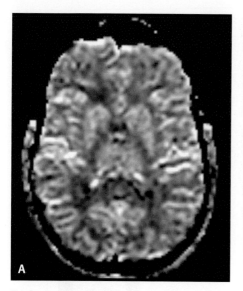 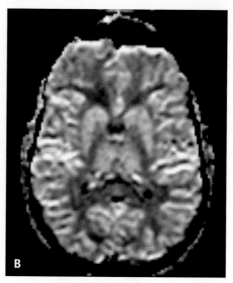

Fig. 8   Dysprosium perfusion imaging.

(**A**) and (**B**). Comparison of 0.2 mmol/kg gado-diamide vs. 0.2 mmol/kg sprodiamide. There is a 30–40% signal drop with sprodiamide, about double that of gadodiamide. (Images are spin echo EPI similar to the protocol described in Table **2**.)

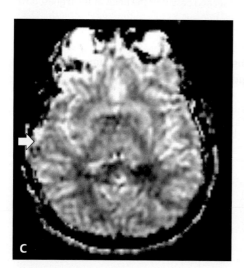 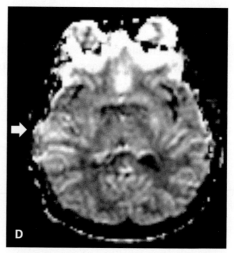

Gadodiamide-based rCBV map   Sprodiamide-based rCBV map

(**C–D**) Note that the resultant CBV maps dem-onstrate higher contrast between gray and white matter, and less heterogeneity in the deep gray matter, indicating decreased noise with the sprodiamide. The arrow highlights the increased rCBV in a tumor.

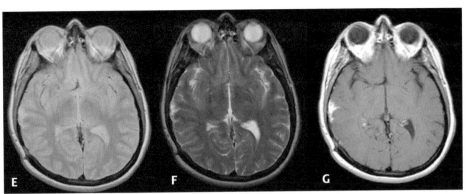

Proton Density   T2-weighted   Post-Gd T1-weighted

8 **(E–G)** Conventional images in a woman with a grade 2 glioma. Note the enhancement indicating blood-brain barrier breakdown. On gadodiamide-based rCBV images (without the correction algorithm) there is decreased rCBV in this area; this is not seen with dysprosium. See also Fig. **54** (p. 114) for another example of dysprosium imaging.

Yet another class of possible future perfusion imaging agents are the iron oxide agents. Superparamagnetic iron oxides (SPIO) exhibit a stronger susceptibility effect than the paramagnetic chelates; however, only few clinical trials investigating the first pass T2 effects of these agents have been performed as yet. The data available describe experiments in animals and preliminary clinical studies. The strong susceptibility effect and small injection volume of iron oxide formulations are advantageous for perfusion MR imaging. However, the toxicity of early formulations has in the past prevented rapid injections of iron oxide formulations in humans. Some work on agents that will be injectable at a bolus rate has been done. For example, the SPIO SH U 555 A (Resovist; Schering AG, Berlin) consists of superparamagnetic iron oxide nanoparticles with a hydrodynamic diameter of 61.1 nm and an iron oxide core of 4.2 nm coated with a carboxydextran shell. The agent is bolus injectable at rates of 4 mL/s and provides small injection volume of ≤ 3 mL at a dose of 16 μmol Fe/kg body weight. The small volume required for injection is advantageous to obtain a compact bolus. The compound allows a stronger reduction in gray and white matter signal intensity (28 and 44%, respectively, with 16 μmol Fe/kg body weight) compared to paramagnetic chelates using T2*-weighted FLASH as has been demonstrated at 1.0 Tesla. Fig. **9** demonstrates perfusion imaging with iron oxide agents.

Gadopentetate dimeglumine at a dose of 0.1 mmol/kg body weight leads to a signal decrease comparable to the dose of 4 μmol Fe/kg body weight [Gd: gray matter 11% and white matter 5% versus Fe: gray matter 13% and white matter 7%]. This indicates the potential of bolus injectable SPIO for dynamic imaging: it could be an improvement in two ways. First, because it appears to cause stronger changes in signal intensity than paramagnetic chelates for a unit dose, improved SNR should be possible. Second, if the

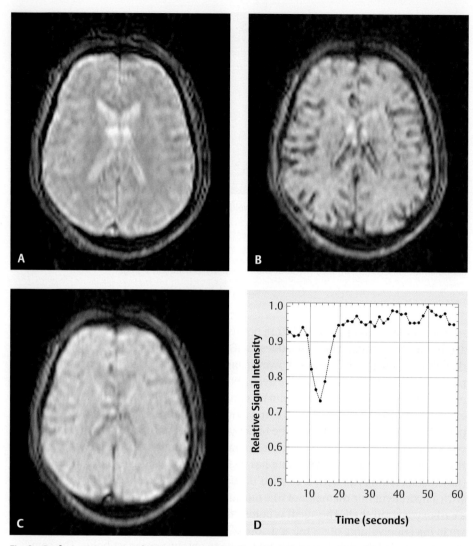

Fig. 9   Perfusion imaging with SPIO at 16 μmol Fe/kg body weight.

Sequential images (**A**) before (upper left), (**B**) during peak signal loss (upper right and lower left) and (**C**) 60 sec (lower right), and normalized signal intensity curves (**D**) following bolus iv administration of SH U 555 A at a dose of 16 μmol Fe/kg body weight. See also Movie Clip ⊙ **6**.

agent is long-lived, then it should be possible to improve SNR for CBV mapping simply by acquiring additional images after the injection of contrast agent and signal averaging. A clinical trial with SPIO is currently under preparation. Future studies have to evaluate whether SPIO are suited to replace paramagnetic chelates for dynamic MR imaging of the brain or heart.

What about non-contrast techniques?

One of the most exciting concepts in MR imaging of blood flow is the possibility to do so without any extrinsic contrast agents. Such approaches typically label the spins of flowing blood in the arteries to make images of flow [25-27]. There are a number of potential theoretical and practical advantages to such arterial spin-labeling techniques, including the possibility of absolute cerebral blood flow measurements. However, in their current formulation these techniques, while promising, are not yet ready to replace contrast-enhanced perfusion MRI. The main reason for this is the superior signal-to-noise ratio of dynamic susceptibility contrast MRI. The contrast-to-noise ratio of gadolinium-based maps of CBF is much greater than ASL-based maps of CBF per unit time. Indeed, ASL maps typically require 5 – 10 minutes or more to create images with even moderate contrast-to-noise ratios. Gadolinium-based approaches, however, require about 1 minute of acquisition time, produce diagnostic-quality images, and in experienced hands are quite reliable. Because of this, the vast majority of perfusion MRI carried out in most institutions is done with contrast agents, and likely will be for at least the next few years while the non-contrast techniques are improved. Nevertheless, such approaches do carry some important benefits. Fig. **10** demonstrates the power of these ASL techniques. While the SNR is noticeably lower, even at 3 T, for a longer imaging time, we believe that with further development ASL will take on a routine clinical role. Areas of active investigation include testing these approaches at low-flow values; some of the key assumptions underlying the potentially quantitative CBF measurements may break down at low blood flow rates. Further testing is essential because such low-flow states are precisely the clinical areas of greatest interest. We look forward to the continued development of these techniques and hope to see more clinical studies performed with them.

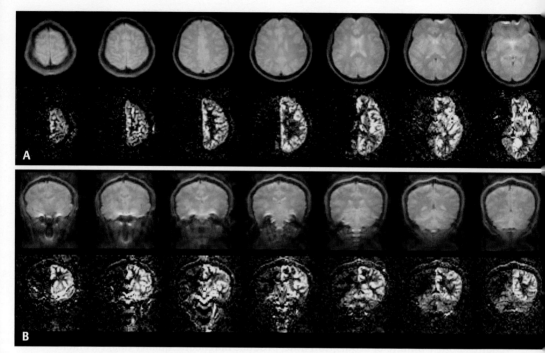

Fig. 10   Arterial spin labeling for measurement of perfusion.

(A) Axial images. Multislice axial control *(top)* and subtraction *(bottom)* images created using a unilateral carotid labeling coil and spin echo EPI (TR/TE/label period/post-label delay 54 s/ 22 ms/3 s/0.5 s, with 7 slices acquired in 500 ms). As expected in the normal brain, perfusion from one carotid artery supplies only the ipsilateral hemisphere. The excellent subtraction of the contralateral hemisphere serves as a demonstration of the elimination of magnetization transfer effects. The images were acquired in 14 min using a TEM head coil.

(B) Coronal multislice control *(top)* and subtraction *(bottom)* images (TR/TE/label period/ post-label delay 54 s/22 ms/3 s/0.5 s, with 7 slices acquired in 500 ms). Note the bright labeling of only the left carotid artery, which can be seen in the third image from anterior. In this subject, some labeling was present in at least one of the vertebral arteries resulting in a partial perfusion signal in the cerebellum. The images were acquired in 14 min using a TEM head coil (from Zaharchuk G, Ledden PJ, Kwong KK, Reese TG, Rosen BR, Wald LL 1999 [137]).

Why use rapid imaging techniques?

Just as a bolus injection is required to best study blood flow, rapid imaging techniques are required to properly time resolve the first pass of the contrast agents. This first pass forms the basis of perfusion imaging. To resolve the first pass a time resolution of at least less than 2 s per slice is mandatory. All current scanners allow for the acquisition of T2*-weighted gradient echo techniques providing a time resolution of < 2 s per image. Such a non-echo planar technique is typically limited to a single slice. Of course, two or three separate injections at a dose of 0.15 or 0.1 mmol gadolinium/kg body weight may be performed to achieve a greater anatomical coverage of the brain (see Fig. **11**). However, such separate injections are typically time consuming and impractical. Instead, the desired multislice capability is provided by echo-planar imaging which requires high performance gradient systems, typically ≥ 15 mT/m. Echo-planar imaging typically provides sequential MR images in less than 100 ms, permitting many slices of the brain to be scanned with a temporal resolution of under 3 seconds. In clinical practice, we recommend the use of echo-planar techniques, since temporal resolution is so important. As shown in Fig. **12**, removing half of the images from a normal study and simulating a lower temporal resolution will degrade the quality of the images one acquires.

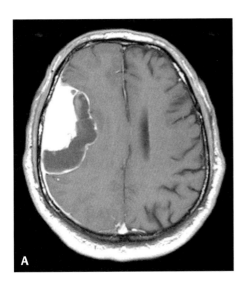

A

Fig. **11**   Repeated injections for greater coverage. Images are from 50-year-old male who underwent three serial perfusion injections.

Post-contrast imaging (**A**) demonstrates an extra-axial mass consistent with a meningioma. The injections were separated by approximately 3 minutes. 0.1 mmol/kg was injected. A "Turbo-FLASH" gradient echo (non-EPI) sequence was used with TR = 32 ms, TE = 22 ms, 64 × 128 matrix, 23 × 23 cm FOV, and slice thickness of 5 mm.

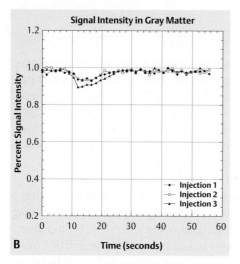

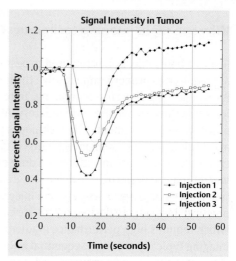

11   The time course from the injections in the gray matter (**B**) is roughly equivalent in each injection. However, due to the disrupted blood brain barrier in the lesion, there is marked enhancement after the first injection that is not present in the later injections (**C**).

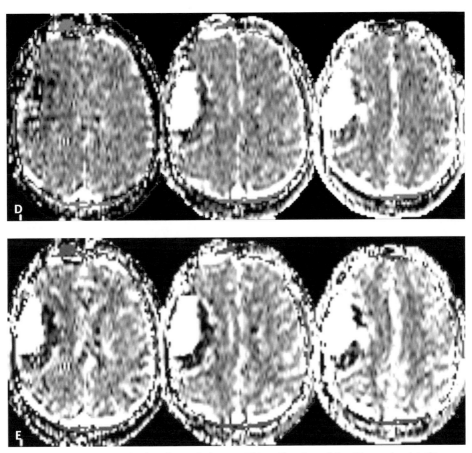

11   The enhancement in the first (lowest) slice presents an artifactually low rCBV (left image, part **D**). However, subsequent images do not show this artifact (center and right images, **D**). This artifact is explained in greater detail in the text (see p. 16 – 20). Corrected rCBV maps, shown in (**E**), do not show this artifact. See also Movie Clips ⊙ **7, 8,** and **9.**

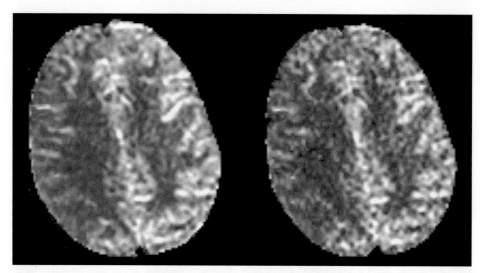

Fig. **12**   The cost of long TR in SNR. On the left is a standard 1.5 TR map of CBF in a patient presenting with symptoms of acute stroke. The right hemisphere perfusion defect is clear. On the left is the same dataset, but subsampled every other image for an effective TR of 3.0 seconds. Note the degradation in image quality, the grainy appearance of the white matter, and the reduced gray-white contrast. The stroke/non-stroke delineation is still possible, but with somewhat reduced confidence.

This may raise the question, how fast is too fast? Is there some rate of image repetition (i.e., TR) at which there is a drawback? Because multislice acquisitions typically push for longer and longer TR values, this question is usually of interest only in the rare instance that only a single slice is of clinical interest. When one is truly interested in sampling the bolus as rapidly as possible (such as in a single-slice acquisition), the optimal repetition time or TR is not just "as short as possible." While minimizing TR would be the correct optimization if one were simply trying to frequently sample the bolus and thereby improve detection, a very short TR (say, less than 500 ms) is not optimal for MR contrast perfusion imaging. Instead, the optimal TR is around 1 second. This is because the trade-off involves not just improvements in SNR with increased sampling frequency, but also decreased sensitivity to T2* effects. As TR gets shorter, the image becomes more T1 weighted, thus producing less sensitivity to T2 effects, and therefore lower-quality perfusion maps. Fig. **13** demonstrates this graphically. We find that in clinical practice, another important trade-off is minimizing the TR versus the number of slices, so that as indicated above we choose a TR of 1.5 seconds and use this to image 10 or more slices.

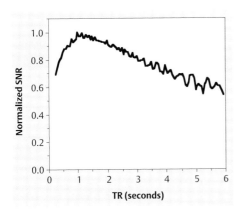

Fig. **13**   The high cost of long TR or of too-short TR. This graph of contrast to noise of CBV maps as a function of TR for spin echo EPI demonstrates that as TR lengthens, the bolus is sampled less efficiently and therefore the contrast to noise decreases. As TR drops below about 800 ms, the acquisition becomes more T1 weighted than T2 weighted, and sensitivity to signal change due to the presence of the contrast agent decreases. Hence, the optimal TR is roughly between 800 and 2200 ms (figure courtesy of R. Weisskoff).

Should I use spin echo or gradient echo EPI?

T2 weighted SE EPI techniques are more specific for the microvasculature than T2* weighted gradient echo imaging techniques. This aspect of susceptibility physics has been demonstrated using simulation studies [17,28], and is illustrated in practice in Fig. **14**. This indicates an important advantage of the SE MRI techniques over other perfusion techniques, including nuclear kinetic studies. The MRI signal changes are weighted by contrast agent in the microvasculature – that is, the capillary bed – rather than in the total vascular space. This is helpful in image generation and interpretation because it brings the dynamic range of the images in to a relevant range. Remember that gray matter has about 4% blood volume, white matter about 2%, and dead tissue or CSF about 0%. Making the distinction between 0, 2, and 4 is easier when there are no voxels with 100% blood volume – such as the large vessels – dominating and therefore obscuring the contrast in the image. This microvascular sensitivity also has important implications in studying neoplastic disorders, due to the role of tumor microvascular angiogenic factors in cancer pathogenesis. This implies that for detection of microvascular perfusion, spin echo techniques provide an increase in specificity, albeit with some loss of signal to noise. We use spin echo imaging almost exclusively, despite its need for a larger dose of contrast agent.

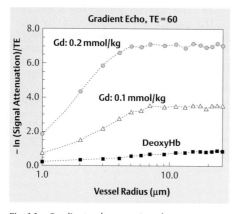
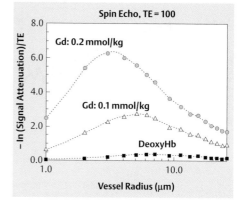

Fig. 14   Gradient echo vs. spin echo.

(**A**) Graphs comparing signal change as a function of susceptibility effect and vessel radius demonstrate relative specificity to small vessels that spin echo acquisitions have compared to gradient echo acquisitions (graphs courtesy of R. Weisskoff and J. Boxerman).

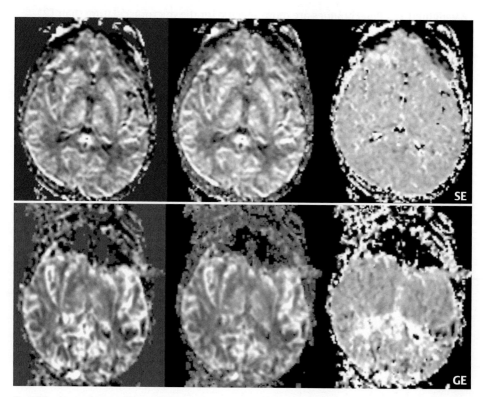

Fig. **14 B**   Legend see p. 35.

Of course, not all users will decide that the microvascular sensitivity is worth the decreased overall sensitivity and/or the additional dose of contrast agent that SE techniques require. For example, in instances where only hemispheric abnormalities might be of interest, gradient echo techniques might suffice. Or, it may be that the particular MR instrument being used does not have adequate image quality with SE EPI but instead does well with GE EPI. Nevertheless, in our experience the boost in image quality for SE is worth the extra effort and/or expense.

What are the detailed typical parameters for perfusion imaging?

Non-EPI Systems

Perfusion studies on conventional systems can be performed with a single section $T2^*$-weighted gradient echo technique. The patient is typically placed in a head coil used for regular clinical imaging. Axial $T2^*$-weighted FLASH images are typically obtained at an FOV of 200–250 mm with a 128 × 64 acquisition matrix and 4–8 mm sections. Typical parameters with a repetition time of 25–35 ms, an echo time of 15–25 ms, a 10–20° flip angle and 1 acquisition provide a time resolution in the order of ≤ 2 s per image. Images are subsequently postprocessed to generate parameter maps.

EPI Systems

Use of an EPI capable system is the preferred approach because of the superior performance. Perfusion studies on systems with echo-planar capability now available for many 0.5–1.5 T systems are also performed with the patient placed in a standard head coil used for regular clinical imaging. Sequential single-shot EPI-SE images are obtained preferably with a "multislice" mode obtained at an FOV of 200–250 mm with a 128 × 64–128 acquisition matrix and 4–8 mm sections. Typical parameters (Table **4**) with a repetition time of 1400–2000 ms and an echo time of 60–75 ms provide a time resolution in the order of 1 s per section. Images are typically obtained for 1 minute to resolve first-pass transit. Images are subsequently postprocessed to generate parameter maps.

◀ **14** **(B)** Images demonstrate the difference in appearance for spin echo (top row) compared to gradient echo images (bottom row). Note the improved gray-white distinction possible on SE images compared with GE images. Cortical vessels are less apparent, allowing more subtle distinctions to be made in the parenchyma. This subject had dental appliances which caused marked susceptibility effects and signal drop out anteriorly on the GE images. Note also that the noise thresholds chosen for computing these maps happen to highlight the greater amount of noise present in gradient echo images. See also Movie Clips ⊙ **10, 11,** and **12**.

Table **4**   Overview of Perfusion MRI Parameters

Parameter	Typical value	Range of values; factors to consider
TR	1500 ms	1000 – 2000 ms; more than 2 seconds and CBF maps become much less useful because of insufficient sampling of the first passage of contrast agent through the brain; if TR is less than 1500 ms then slice count drops below 10.
TE	65 ms	50 – 80 ms; the balance is between T2 and T2* weighting and insufficient signal because of T2 decay. For a given dose, the ideal amount of signal drop is about 1/e. Typically this means the TE should be about the same as the T2 (roughly 50 ms or so). See [17] for more detailed information.
FOV	20 cm × 20 cm	20 cm × 20 cm to 24 cm × 24 cm; however, this is widely variable depending on the needs of the system. We have also used 20 × 40 with good results (with a corresponding 128 × 256 readout).
Matrix	128 × 128	64 × 64 to 256 × 256; multishot EPI is probably not a good idea since the contrast will pass through too quickly to be seen well with multishot techniques. Also, if the matrix gets too fine then SNR in each voxel becomes limited. This may be able to change as TE values get shorter and more powerful contrast agents are available.
Slice thickness	6 mm	5 to 10 mm. Again, SNR limits this some. Thicker slices can certainly be used but with the drawback of volume averaging. For screening studies, 10 slices at 10 mm each is certainly enough to cover much of the brain and will have excellent SNR.
Interslice gap	1 mm or interleaved	0 – 10 mm. On some systems a gap is necessary to reduce crosstalk. On the other hand, a large gap is an easy way to increase coverage for screening purposes.
Number of repeated images at each slice	45	32 – 80. While the bolus itself may only be visible on a dozen or fewer images, acquisition of an adequate baseline is essential. Baselines are best characterized with many images; one simulation study found that 50 or more images (in the baseline alone!) provided the best improvement in SNR [23]. Many clinical systems are limited to 512 images, and so for 11 slices no more than 46 images per slice can be obtained. This limits the baseline to about 15 images.
Disabled acquisitions	2	0 – 4. Remember that with a TR of 1.5 seconds or so, there will be some T1 effects. These manifest themselves as decreasing signal intensity after the first image. (See Movie Clip ⊙ **14**). One way to avoid the problems this can cause is to simply tell the postprocessing software to ignore the first two images when calculating perfusion maps. However, if the acquisition is limited to 512 images, then ignoring the first two images is giving up potentially important data. One can avoid this problem by instructing the scanner to acquire two or three EPI images but not actually reconstruct the data. These are sometimes called "disabled acquisitions".

Table **4** Exploration parameters for perfusion imaging *(continuation)*

Parameter	Typical value	Range of values; factors to consider
Number of slices	11	5–20. More slices typically means a longer TR, and too long a TR hurts both steady-state SNR (per unit time) and the sampling of the dynamic bolus. We typically put as many slices in a TR of 1.5 as our machine will let us.
Total imaging time	TR × number of repeated images = 45 × 1.5 = 68 seconds	30 seconds to 3 minutes; depends on the number of images at each slice and the TR.
Time of injection	10 seconds after imaging begins	5–30 seconds. Remember that it takes about 10 seconds to pass through the lungs, through the heart, and up in to the brain. In addition, the bolus has a duration of 5 to 10 seconds, and it is widened by passage through the lungs. The longer you can wait to collect more baseline images, the better (see above), but if too many baseline images are collected then the bolus might be missed, or the signal change after the bolus has passed might be missed.
Amount of contrast	0.2 mmol/kg (e.g., 40 mL for a 100 kg person)	0.05 to 0.4 mmol/kg (e.g., 40 mL for a 100 kg person). Basically, the more contrast agent injected, the better the SNR. However, 0.1 mmol/kg can be visualized at 1.5 T and appears to be adequate at 3.0 T.
Rate of injection	5 mL/second	2–5 mL/second. Too slow a bolus will preclude effective T2 and T2* changes because the concentration will be diminished. However, if the diameter of the iv cannula is too small (less than 18–20 gauge), the rate must be turned down to prevent leakage.
Amount of saline flush	25 mL	10 to 30 mL. The goal is to flush the gadolinium out of the arm, out of the lungs, and into the brain. Once it reaches the heart this is largely done by the heart.
Rate of saline flush	5 mL/second	5 mL/second. Same as above.
Size of iv catheter	18 gauge or larger	22 gauge to 14 gauge. We place an iv line in the antecubital fossa. We use an 18 gauge needle not because a 20 gauge cannot handle 5 mL/second but because the use of the larger cannula helps remind the person inserting the iv line that a large vein needs to be used. We have used central lines; in cases where only a 22 gauge needle can be used we may drop the injection rate to 2 mL/s.

Can you tell me more about the optimum contrast agent dose?

The dose of contrast agent used is important. Simply put, larger doses provide a greater signal change; greater signal change typically means better perfusion images, up to a point. If the signal decrease is greater than about 40–50% (more precisely, 1/e), additional Gd leads to a decrease in quality rather than increase [23]. Since for SE EPI, 0.1 mmol/kg leads to an average drop of about 10–15%, for the most part this upper limit is not reached in routine practice. Indeed, although doses of 0.1 mmol/kg of Gd can be used at 1.5 T, several studies have found that higher doses of 0.2–0.3 mmol Gd/kg body weight to be significantly superior. The dose of 0.3 mmol Gd/kg body weight is the highest approved dose which can be used, although some physicians (including ourselves) have given higher doses without evidence of side effects. The differentiation of gray and white matter, as well as the overall quality of CBV maps, improves with increasing the dose as shown in Tables **5** and **6**. In some cases, larger doses allow shorter TEs to be used with a resulting improvement in SNR.

Table **5**   Dose-dependent quality of perfusion maps: differentiation of gray and white matter[1]

Dose	No %	Equivocal %	Good %	Excellent %
0.1 mmol Gd				
normal	54.5	18.2	27.3	
diseased	60.0	20.0	20.0	
0.2 mmol Gd				
normal	20.0	40.0	30.0	10.0
diseased	20.0	20.0	20.0	40.0
0.3 mmol Gd				
normal	10.5	36.8	42.1	10.5
diseased		60.0	40.0	
0.4 mmol Gd				
normal		15.0	25.0	60.0
diseased			33.3	66.7
0.5 mmol Gd				
normal		20.0	60.0	20.0
diseased		33.3	33.3	33.3

[1] Five different doses of gadobutrol were injected at a desired injection rate of 5 mL/s in 80 patients with a power injector through 18–22 g iv lines in 80 patients with unilateral carotid stenosis and/or stroke in the anterior circulation. Acquisition parameters include: TR = 32 ms, TE = 22 ms, 64 × 128 matrix, 230 mm FOV, single slice, 1.27 minute imaging window, 1.0 Tesla Siemens Impact Expert system. The table shows dose-dependent differentiation of gray and white matter from 0.1 to 0.5 mmol of gadobutrol per kg body weight. Determination was made by two neuroradiologists in consensus. The gray and white matter differentiation increases with increasing dose to 0.4 mmol gadobutrol per kg body weight. Results in diseased hemispheres show a stronger dose dependency than in normal hemispheres. These data imply that the standard clinical dose of 0.1 mmol gadobutrol per kg body weight (or any other Gd-based agent) might not provide reliable results with this imaging technique.

Table **6**   Dose-dependent quality of perfusion maps: identifying lesions[1]

Dose	Inadequate %	Adequate %	Good %	Excellent %
0.1 mmol Gd				
normal	72.7	18.2	9.1	
diseased	80.0		20.0	
0.2 mmol Gd				
normal	40.0	40.0	10.0	10.0
diseased	20.0	20.0	40.0	20.0
0.3 mmol Gd				
normal	21.1	36.8	31.6	10.5
diseased	40.0		40.0	20.0
0.4 mmol Gd				
normal	5.0		60.0	35.0
diseased				100.0
0.5 mmol Gd				
normal		20.0	60.0	20.0
diseased		33.3	33.3	33.3

[1] Five different doses of gadobutrol were injected at a desired injection rate of 5 mL/s in 80 patients with unilateral carotid stenosis and/or stroke in the anterior circulation. The table shows dose-dependent quality of CBV maps from 0.1 – 0.5 mmol of gadobutrol per kg body weight as graded by blinded readers. The dose of 0.4 mmol gadobutrol per kg body weight produces the best quality of CBV maps for the acquisition parameters in this study (acquisition and interpretation parameters were identical to those described in Table **5**). Results in diseased hemispheres show a stronger dose dependency than normal hemispheres. Again, these data imply that the standard clinical dose of 0.1 mmol gadobutrol per kg body weight may not provide reliable results. One reason for this might be that in disease states, the delivery of contrast agent may be reduced. This means that a dose that might be adequate for analysis of normal brain might prove inadequate in the face of pathology.

Do I need a power injector? How do I use it?

Use of a MR-compatible power injector (see Fig. **5**, p. 16) facilitates a standardized injection; this helps obtain comparable and reliable data. The MR power injector allows flushing with saline before the injection at low rate (1 – 2 mL per minute) that helps to keep the venous access open. In addition, the system can provide a bolus of saline, which will advance the contrast agent column through the veins of the upper arm and shoulder into the superior vena cava and heart without any delay following the contrast bolus. The benefits of standardization, ease of use, and ability to keep the vein open during the scanning prior to perfusion MR all weigh in favor of the injector. Furthermore, the injector can provide a high rate of injection, something that is difficult to achieve manually. Of course, the rate that is prescribed is often not the rate that is delivered, as shown in Figs. **15** and **16**. This is because the tubing and size of the iv cannula can slow the passage of the contrast agent, in addition to the viscosity of the agent itself. Nevertheless, these power injectors have gained popularity because of their ability to overcome or at least standardize a solution to many of these issues.

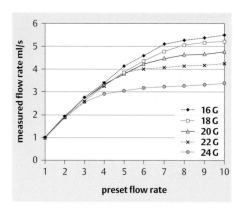

Fig. **15**   Relationship of flow rates and iv lines. The relationship of preset flow rates and measured flow rates when using different iv lines is shown for gadopentetate dimeglumine at room temperature injected with a flow-controlled power injector (Spectris, MEDRAD Inc, Inola, PA) (courtesy of T. Allkemper).

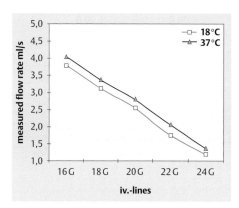

Fig. **16**   Injection rates at room temperature and body temperature. The relationship of measured flow rates and different iv lines is shown for gadopentetate dimeglumine at room temperature versus body temperature. Injections were performed with a pertubent-controlled power injector (Ullrich AG, FRG). The flow rate increases by less than 0.5 mL/s following warming of the contrast agent (courtesy of T. Allkemper).

The size of the iv line is important to maintain a stable flow rate. Fig. **15** shows that a preset flow rate of 5 mL/s with a flow-controlled power injector (Spectris, MEDRAD Inc, Inola, PA) translates into a real flow rate of 4 mL/s, but only when using 16–22 g iv lines. Results with other gadolinium chelates are identical and warming of the contrast agent to room temperature accelerates injections by less than 0.5 mL/s (Fig. **16**).

We recommend placing the iv lines in an antecubital vein for reasons discussed in Table **4** (p. 36).

How do I perform a manual injection?

In case a power injector is not available a manual injection can be performed. Manual injection works best if it is standardized by using a dedicated tubing set. An example of such a standardized tubing set is shown in Fig. 17. As with the power injection, we recommend placing the iv lines in an antecubital vein, and also the assembly of a system to allow injection of saline after the injection of contrast agent. This is typically accomplished with a stopcock valve or a bifurcated "y" check valve system attached to two syringes: one filled with saline, and one filled with contrast agent. The person doing the injection goes into the room with the patient before the scan, attaches the injection system, and then watches the countdown clock for the proper time to inject. By using as much force as possible, the contrast agent can typically be injected at 3 to 5 mL/second; there is, however, a short delay while moving from the use of one syringe to use of the other. While the image quality can be as good as with a power injector, reproducibility and reliability is probably lower.

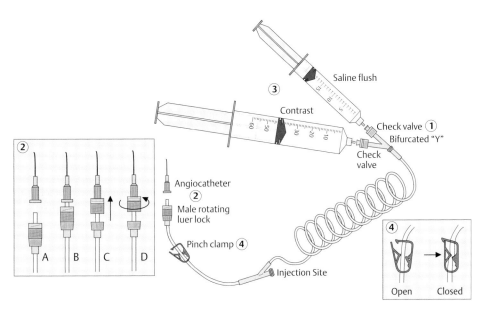

Fig. 17   Standardized tubing set for intravenous Infusions (Smart Set, Topspins, www.topspins. com). A 2 meter length of coiled tubing has two injections sites with checkflow valves (1) to permit simultaneous attachment of a 60 ml contrast syringe and a 20 or 30 ml saline flush syringe (3). The automatic check-flow valve system allows immediate switching from the contrast infusion to saline flush. This avoids having a gap in the middle of the bolus which can degrade image quality.

Is the injection volume important?

The injection volume increases with increasing doses for a given concentration of Gd-based medium. For example, increasing the dose for a 75 kg subject from 0.1 mmol Gd/kg body weight to 0.3 mmol Gd/kg body weight increases the injection volume from 14 to 42 mL. (These figures are for 0.5 molar gadolinium chelates, the typical concentration). Giving a constant injection rate of 5 mL/s provided by a power injector, the injection time increases also by a factor of 3 (from 3 to 9 s) spreading the bolus equally over more heart cycles. This means that the bolus transit time also increases and it takes more time to reach the maximum signal decrease. This increased bolus width might blur the slight differences in arrival time between voxels. Therefore, by just giving more contrast agent to generate better perfusion images we may run into volume limitations. While there is currently no way around this problem in most countries, one solution that has been developed is to increase the concentration of Gd. More highly concentrated gadolinium chelates such as gadobutrol (currently approved for use in at least one European country) enable an increase in dose to 0.3 mmol Gd/kg body weight (0.3 mmol Gd/kg body weight = 21 ml) with less of an impact on the bolus width as measured by time to peak signal change. Examples of the increase of time-to-peak at doses > 0.3 mmol Gd/kg body weight are shown in Fig. **18**. Therefore smaller volumes such as are possible with dysprosium-based or iron-based agents would be desirable.

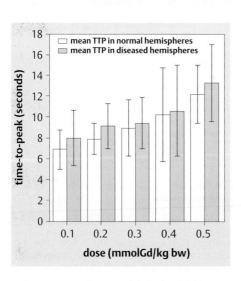

Fig. **18** Time-to-peak as a function of dose and volume. Five different doses of gadobutrol were injected at a desired injection rate of 5 mL/s with a power injector through 18–22 g iv lines in 80 patients with unilateral carotid stenosis and/or stroke in the anterior circulation. The graph shows a significant time-to-peak increase with increasing doses/volumes ≥ 0.4 mmol Gd/kg body weight. Error bars show standard deviation in the region of interest.

Is field strength important?

Susceptibility effects on T2 and T2* change approximately linearly with field strength. Therefore, susceptibility effects are more pronounced at high field (1.5 T, 3.0 T, or higher) than at mid field (1.0 T) or low field ($\leq$ 0.5 T) systems. An increase in contrast agent dose can compensate for this decrease at low field strengths and perfusion studies are therefore not restricted to high field. Several studies at 0.5 and 1 T have demonstrated the feasibility of perfusion imaging at field strengths < 1.5 T. On the other hand, by going to very high field such as 3.0 T, the effect per dose of agent increases and therefore the SNR increases. This can be traded off for a lower dose and equivalent SNR, or the improvement in SNR can allow thinner slices or smaller voxels, depending on the choice of the radiologist.

How do I postprocess perfusion images?

Postprocessing is essential to creating perfusion images. A variety of approaches to postprocessing has been proposed, but for the sake of simplicity, we will focus on a small family of image types: CBV, CBF, and MTT. One hindrance to the routine use of perfusion is the lack of postprocessing tools from the manufacturers; fortunately, this is currently changing. Support from equipment manufacturers will obviate problems of file formats, header information, archiving, etc. and instead let the user focus on the clinical issues.

Overview

Typically, functional parameter images can be generated quite rapidly once the initial EPI images are available. CBV, CBF, MTT, and other parameter images can then be analyzed and compared with the dynamic images to search for disease abnormalities. Most of the algorithms that produce these functional images require the user to input a few key data, such as which image the bolus begins to arrive at, and which image represents the end of the first pass of the contrast agent through the brain. Other information, such as the TR, can be obtained from the image header. For maps of CBF that require the extra data set known as the arterial input function, the user will be required to choose an appropriate set of voxels to extract the arterial input function from. This section of this book will discuss how these decisions are to be made.

Step 0: Before you start

Before attempting to make maps or do meaningful analysis on a perfusion MRI data set, it is wise to examine the raw data to ensure its freedom from major artifacts such as gross patient motion, scanner failure, lack of delivery of contrast agent, or any number of other technical flaws that can preclude useful analysis. Movie Clip ⊙ **13** demonstrates an example of a case where the patient moved just as the bolus of contrast was injected, rendering the baseline images worthless (unless some type of motion correction algorithm is employed). Such artifacts can be common and successful routine perfusion imaging requires establishing protocols and routines to reduce their occurrence, such as coaching patients about what to expect.

Step 1: The initial parameter of concentration versus time

After injection, the concentration of contrast agent in a given voxel varies with time. The log of the signal measured on MRI reflects the approximately linear relationship between the change observed in the T2 rate, $\Delta(1/T2) = \Delta R2$, and the concentration of Gd. Therefore we can estimate the concentration of Gd – at least in relative terms – by measuring the percent signal change from baseline. Within some limiting range, therefore, we can measure the contrast agent's concentration in tissue as a function of time (the so-called "concentration-versus-time" curve) by mapping tissue signal loss dynamically over time as shown in Fig. **19**. This requires some type of image display software that treats the 40 + images in a given slice as a large but single chunk of data. Thinking about this data set as a movie at each slice may be helpful, since from now on what goes on in each slice is a dynamic event. (Reviewing Movie Clip ⊙ **1** where the data from Fig. **19** were obtained may be helpful.)

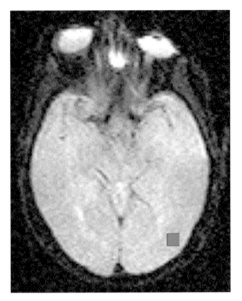 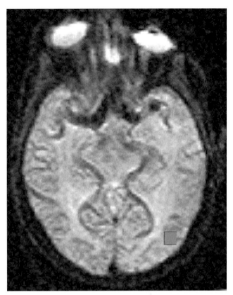

Fig. 19 Plot of signal versus time for a region of interest in normal gray matter (data are taken from Movie Clip ⊙ **1**.

(A) Region of interest at baseline.   **(B)** Region of interest at peak signal change.

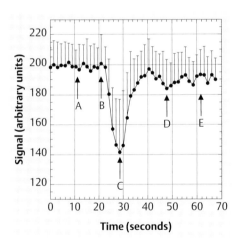

(C) Graph of signal change over time in region of interest. Arrows point out baseline A, arrival B), peak signal change C, recirculation peak D, and slight drop in post-contrast baseline E compared to pre-contrast A.

Step 2: Analyzing the curve

Before we discuss how to further process the data, it would be useful to spend some time looking at a sample data set and identifying some of its major features. Well-performed perfusion data sets have a steady baseline (Arrow A in Fig. **19**) followed by a clear-cut arrival of the contrast bolus (Arrow B). The signal drop is typically 20–30% or more (Arrow C), has a relatively narrow time course, and often a second smaller drop in signal can be seen as the bolus recirculates (Arrow D). Finally, the intravascular contrast has some residual susceptibility effects, causing a slight drop in signal (a few percent) compared to pre-baseline (Arrow E). A technologist or radiologist can quickly determine whether or not a given examination was of adequate quality by examining the signal versus time curve with a suitable ROI drawn. If there was extensive patient motion, or if the bolus never arrived, or if the scanner had technical problems, all of these issues will be at once obvious when looking at the curves. Just as in MRA, where analysis of the raw data solves many problems, analysis of the curves with perfusion MRI can make a big difference.

Remember that the signal drop versus time curve can be easily turned into a concentration versus time curve by taking the negative log of the signal change, as shown in Figs. **20** and **21**.

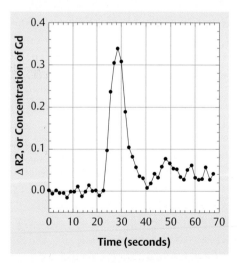

Fig. **20**   Conversion of data from Fig. **19**. Instead of plotting signal intensity versus time, the data are converted to a change in 1/T2, or R2, versus time.

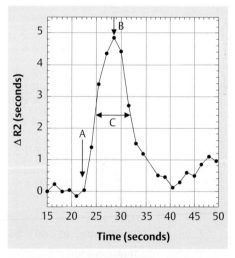

Fig. **21**   Focus on a portion of Fig. **20**. Arrow A points to the arrival time, arrow B to the peak signal change, and arrow C to the width of the curve at half its maximum.

Step 3: Creating the maps: CBV

Cerebral blood volume is one of the most robust and simple perfusion maps to create. Mathematical integration of the area under the ΔR2 curve in each voxel produces values that are proportional to the CBV in each voxel, similar to standard tracer experiments used in nuclear medicine. To create these maps, an algorithm only needs to know where to calculate the baseline. Once the user inputs where the baseline begins and ends, then a baseline can be calculated, and the computer can calculate ΔR2 at each point in time using the formula

$$\Delta R2 = \frac{-\ln(S/S_0)}{TE}$$

One then integrates the area underneath this curve to calculate blood volume:

$$CBV \approx \int_0^\infty \Delta R2(t)$$

Note that this formula indicates integrating from 0 to infinity; of course we do not scan any patient infinitely long (although it may feel that way to some subjects). Instead, what this means is that for as long as we do scan, post-contrast images will be CBV-weighted. This means that we do not typically need to specify when the bolus is no longer present; instead, we choose to integrate until the end of the acquisition data. This is because as long as contrast agent is present in the vasculature, it will change the signal in a voxel proportional to its concentration. The practical meaning of this is that as long as the contrast agent stays inside the capillaries, there is no reason not to perform the integration to the end of the scan. This can be seen from Fig. **19**; while there is not as much signal change at Arrow E as there is at Arrow C, there still is signal change, and that signal change will be proportional to the amount of contrast in that voxel. So, adding the data from images toward the end of the acquisition will only improve the SNR of the CBV map. This is *not* the case if the BBB is leaky; in this case one will have competing effects from T2 and T1 effects of the Gd (as described above). In such cases, one may choose to end the integration before the end of the acquisition. Whether one chooses to use the integration software that uses the post-bolus data, or chooses to end integration at the bolus depends on the severity of the BBB breakdown, acquisition parameters, and other factors that may be best determined via trial and error.

One approach to avoiding recirculation artifacts is to fit a curve to the observed time course data at each voxel (or group of voxels). The mathematical formula usually chosen for curve fitting is a gamma variate. In our experience, at high resolution (e.g., 128 × 128 over 20 cm FOV] such curve fitting is detrimental to the overall image quality (as measured with SNR) compared to simple numerical integration [23]. As a result, we use numerical integration routinely.

In summary, to create CBV maps one needs to teach the software where the baseline is (beginning and end). The bolus is assumed to arrive at the end of the baseline, and CBV maps can be improved by integrating until the end of the acquisition unless there is a leaky BBB. If a leaky BBB is suspected or known to exist (from, say, looking at the post-Gd T1 weighted images) then one may wish to curtail integration right at the end of the first bolus, well before Arrow D in the figure, to minimize the BBB breakdown effects.

Step 4: Creating the maps: CBF

Creating CBF maps involves an additional step of specifying an arterial input function. The arterial input function (AIF) is simply another tissue-versus-time curve. That is, it is simply another data set, or list of numbers, that provides information about the timing of the contrast agent through an artery that feeds the tissue of interest. It is typically determined by placing some regions of interest near a major vessel such as the MCA. Why is this AIF needed? The standard equation for flow measurement ends up describing the relationship between the concentration of a tracer in a volume of interest (VOI) and the arterial input of the tracer, $C_a(t)$:

$$C_{VOI}(t) = F_t \int_0^t C_a(\tau)R(t - \tau)d\tau$$

In this equation, F_t is tissue flow and $R(t)$ is the vascular *residue function,* describing the fraction of tracer still present in the vascular bed of the VOI at time t after injection of a unit impulse of tracer in its feeding vessel. We can fit for $R(t)$, but only if we know $C_a(t)$. Fortunately, because the MCA is a relatively large vessel and in the imaging plane, we can get an estimate of $C_a(t)$ by examining voxels near the MCA. One might ask, why not voxels *in* the MCA (rather than near the MCA)? The reason for this is actually related to the reason why quantitative CBF is so difficult with gadolinium-based MR. One of the fundamental assumptions about tracer kinetics is that the signal change is related in a known manner to the amount of contrast agent present in the voxel. While this is true in the brain parenchyma, this is *not* true in the MCA. The MCA, for example, already has a low signal due to flow effects; the passage of Gd through this may cause a further drop, but this is not proportional. Hence, if we want to get an estimate of the flow of contrast agent through the MCA, we look at the voxels just *outside* the MCA. These voxels will be affected by the passage either because of blooming of the susceptibility and/or because of the passage of contrast agent out of the perforating arteries. Additional reasons why quantitative CBF is not yet possible from MCA measurements include the well-known angular dependence of susceptibility-induced signal change: the orientation of the vessel with respect to the magnetic field will cause some change in the susceptibility effects. This is the basis of so-called magic angle spinning, and is a major reason for the lack of correlation between signal change in the large vessels and concentration. Finally, the graphs above in Fig. **14A** (p. 34) document that the sensitivity to signal change is related to vessel size, such that the signal change in the MCA for a given amount of Gd is not the same in large vessels as it is in small vessels.

While we hope to overcome each of these problems and finally obtain true quantitative CBF measurements, for now our conservative opinion is that this is not yet possible. Hence, our images are termed relative CBF (rCBF) and relative CBV (rCBV).

In spite of all of these potential complications, creating CBF maps is actually quite simple from the user's point of view. The computer algorithm needs only two additional pieces of information. First, the ROI containing the AIF must be selected. Fig. **22** shows an example of a typical AIF chosen from near the MCA. Note that the AIF ROI is apparently *outside* the MCA when no contrast agent has been administered, but appears to be *inside* the MCA at the peak of the concentration curve. Note also, from Fig. **22 C**, that the AIF typically has a much greater decline in signal than the tissue concentration curve and therefore a larger $\Delta R2$, as well as a narrower and earlier time course. This greater $\Delta R2$ is shown in Fig. **22 D**. All of these features are consistent with a normal arterial input function. Movie Clip ⊙ **14** highlights a magnified version of the susceptibility effect we are seeking to measure when we choose an AIF. In Movie Clip ⊙ **14**, the same type of susceptibility "blooming" occurs, but because the vessel is larger the effects are more visible.

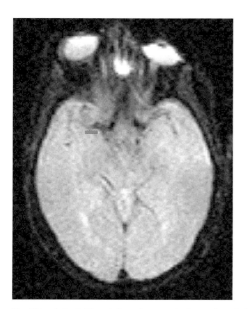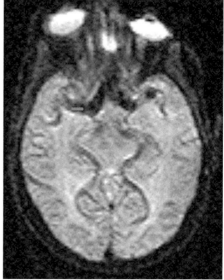

Fig. **22**   Arterial input function, again from data in Movie Clip ⊙ **1**.

(**A**) Region of interest on baseline image. Note that the region of interest is outside the flow void of the right middle cerebral artery.

(**B**) Region of interest on the peak signal change image. Note that now the region of interest, which has not moved, appears inside the flow void of the middle cerebral artery. This is due to signal change from the contrast agent.

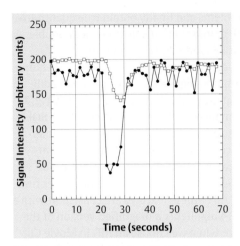

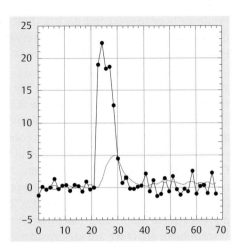

22 (**C**) Plot of signal versus time in the arterial input function region of interest. Also plotted as a dashed line connecting open squares is the same signal versus time intensity curve shown in Fig. **19 C**, now rescaled to fit the same axis as the AIF data.

22 (**D**) Conversion of the time course plots in part C to change in R2 versus time (analogous to Fig. **20**). Note the larger signal change in the AIF, consistent with the higher concentration of Gd in the peri-MCA area than in the capillary bed of the gray matter.

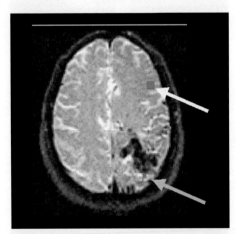

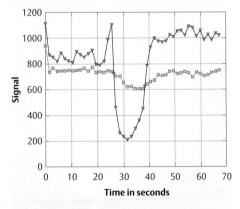

22 (**E**) Susceptibility effects during first pass inside a vessel. A region of interest in frontal gray matter (blue, corresponding to the square points in the graph) shows a roughly 20% signal drop during the first pass of the contrast agent through the tissue. However, a region of interest placed at the parietal lobe (blue, with gray arrow, and signal corresponding to the triangle points in the graph) shows a larger signal drop,

at least 70%. This is because of the larger susceptibility effect of the contrast inside the capillaries. Also of note is the drop in signal during the first two or three images, where steady-state T1 effects are taking place. This is because the TR of 1.5 s leads to some saturation of the images. In other video clips, the first two images are not included, or else the images were not acquired. See also Movie Clip ⊙ **14**.

Once the AIF is selected, the only other thing the algorithm needs to know is when the first pass of contrast agent through the tissue has finished. This is necessary to prevent disturbances from the recirculation peak. With these two pieces of information, CBF maps can then be created.

One question that may arise for advanced users is which AIF to choose. Should one choose the normal MCA, or the abnormal MCA? What about choosing the PCA for posterior regions of the brain? The answers to these questions are still under active investigation. We typically choose the AIF for the region of clinical interest, that is, the area to which symptoms may be attributable. If there is more than one area, we on occasion make multiple sets of CBF and MTT images, particularly because much of the map creation is automated and can be done quickly.

Step 5: Creating the maps: MTT and other timing maps

This is actually the easiest map of all once the other two are created, because by the central volume theorem, CBF = CBV/MTT. Hence, one can create MTT maps by dividing CBV by CBF. It is worth noting that MTT is often mistakenly thought of as the width of the tissue-concentration curve, the measurement corresponding to what is labeled C on Fig. **21** (p. 46). However, as pointed out by Weisskoff et al. [9], this is not really the MTT, although it still may be a useful parameter. Instead, what is labeled as C in $\Delta R2$ with arrows is actually better termed "full width at half maximum" or FWHM. A simple way to understand why FWHM is not MTT is to consider what would happen if the identical flow and volume were present, and the same amount of contrast agent administered, but a different arterial input function were used, say, because of a slower injection rate, or because of carotid stenosis. In such a case, the FWHM would change even though CBV and CBF did not.

While FWHM is not the same as MTT, that does not mean that it is not a useful value. Indeed, there are a number of other "time" maps that can be useful, depending on the clinical setting. These have been simpler to implement computationally, and therefore have gained quite a bit of acceptance in various forms. These include maps of the arrival of the bolus (arrow A in Fig. **21**, p. 46), the time of the peak signal change (arrow B in Fig. **21**), or sometimes the time from the start of the injection to the half maximum value (the left arrow of Arrows marked C in Fig. **21**). Because acute stroke typically causes both changes in the local arterial input function as well as decreased CBF, a map of the delay in the arrival of blood to the area of injury often highlights the hemodynamic change. The concern is that such approaches can be overly sensitive, and may not take into account chronic change.

A good example of this technical problem can be seen below in the section on stroke imaging, and in particular Fig. **37** (p. 77). In a case where there is unilateral vessel stenosis, the timing maps can be abnormal for the whole hemisphere, even when little or no tissue is at risk. Deconvolving the tissue concentration versus time curve with the arterial input function can compensate (at least partially) for such problems.

What advanced techniques may become important in the future?

Compensation for delay and dispersion

In an ideal scenario, each voxel would be treated in a completely independent fashion. That would mean that in addition to looking at the tissue signal versus time curve on a voxel-by-voxel basis, each voxel would have its own appropriately determined AIF. For example, the AIF for voxels in the occipital lobe is likely to be different than the AIF for voxels in the frontal lobe. How might this be accomplished? This is an area of active research, but improvements in these areas are likely to be highly relevant to clinical practice since the false positives and false negatives should be reduced by such an approach. Other physiologists have classified these changes in the local AIF as "delay" and "dispersion." Delay is the slow-down in arrival of the contrast agent without any drop in CBF. This might occur if the patient has a bypass graft or other change in the length of the vessel in one side versus another. Fig. 23 depicts this in cartoon fashion. Dispersion is the "spreading" of the bolus that might occur as the bolus passes through a stenosis, also depicted in Fig. 23. Mathematical approaches to dealing with both of these issues have been developed; it is likely that future versions of perfusion postprocessing software will incorporate such approaches.

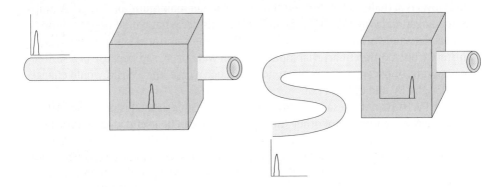

Fig. 23   Delay and dispersion.

(A) A cartoon of the injection of contrast. The small time course graph shows the input of tracer, and the graph on the gray box indicates what measurement in the idealized voxel demonstrates. This part of the cartoon displays the expected pattern of measurement.

(B) Delay. When there is a longer pathway to the voxel relative to the voxel in part A, then the contrast is delayed. Measurement of the arrival time or the time of the peak signal change would highlight this delay.

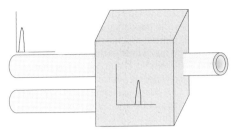

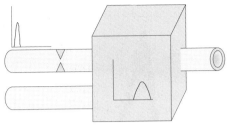

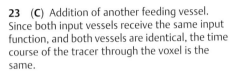

23 (**C**) Addition of another feeding vessel. Since both input vessels receive the same input function, and both vessels are identical, the time course of the tracer through the voxel is the same.

23 (**D**) Stenosis in one of the feeding vessels. This causes dispersion of the contrast agent, and broadening of the tracer curve. This might not be associated with decreased volume or decreased flow, but can be an independent phenomenon.

Flow heterogeneity

The flow in a voxel is actually the average of flows in the many vessels contained in that voxel, since many capillaries are contained even in a small voxel. Indeed, a number of investigators now realize that within a given sample of brain tissue, there is not a single flow value but a distribution of flow values. Laser Doppler and other methods have suggested that there is considerable heterogeneity of flow in the normal cerebral circulation, particularly in the capillary bed. Fig. **24** demonstrates measured flow distributions in normal volunteers, and indicates that there is a distribution of flows around the mean CBF ($f = 1.0$) [29]. Furthermore, as blood flow drops due to hypocapnia or decreased perfusion pressure, this heterogeneity decreases, and the flow becomes more homogeneous. This homogenization may be an effort to increase the efficiency of oxygen and glucose transfer [30,31]. This increase in homogeneity presumably reflects an autoregulatory mechanism [32,33]. Measuring such heterogeneity in a variety of clinical settings (e.g., stroke, brain tumors) should be useful because it could serve as a marker of at least three physiological phenomena. First, an increase in homogeneity (or drop in flow heterogeneity) indicates both the need for autoregulation and the persistence of autoregulatory function. This would serve as an indicator that tissue was threatened enough to need autoregulatory mechanisms to begin, yet still viable enough to invoke such autoregulatory mechanisms. This is shown in Fig. **25**. Second, a severe blood flow drop with a lack of homogenization might indicate that autoregulation was no longer possible, and that tissue was now severely – and possibly irreversibly – compromised. Third, an increase in the disorganization of vessels, and therefore an increase in flow heterogeneity, may be associated with angiogenesis, as shown in Fig. **26**. These techniques may allow further characterization of microvascular physiology.

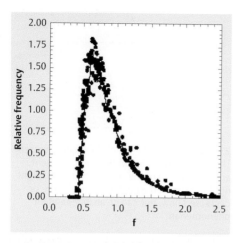

Fig. **24** Heterogeneity of flow as measured in humans [29]. The frequency of each flow measurement is plotted as a function of relative flow (f = 1.0 is the mean flow in the area of measurement.). For example, the graph shows that the most likely flow is approximately ⅔ that of the mean CBF. Many capillaries, however, with just under mean CBF, and some voxels with as much as 2.5 times mean CBF (figure courtesy of L. Østergaard).

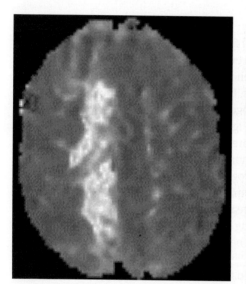

Fig. **25** Drop in flow heterogeneity in acute stroke.

(A) Mean transit time image from same patient as in Fig. **2** (p. 6).

(B) Map of the width of the flow heterogeneity curve in colorized form plotted on top of CBF. Note that only some of the areas of MTT abnormality show a drop in flow heterogeneity. The color scale is arbitrary. Blue arrows point out foci of extreme decreases in flow heterogeneity; compare to figure **35 (D)**.

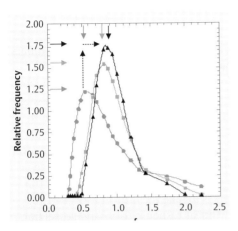

25 (**C**) Analysis of regions of interest in three areas depicted in A. This is a plot of the distribution of the slope of the values in the residue function. Blue is normal brain, with the expected shape, similar to Fig. **24**. Grey and black are two other areas that depict abnormal shifts in flow, with narrowing of the overall curve shape. This narrowing means there is a decrease in the spread of values of CBF, that is, an increased homogeneity. This is the same thing as a decrease in the heterogeneity of the flow.

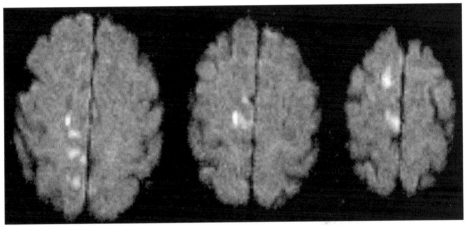

25 (**D**) Follow-up images depict infarction in the same areas where flow heterogeneity was most abnormal (figure courtesy of L. Østergaard).

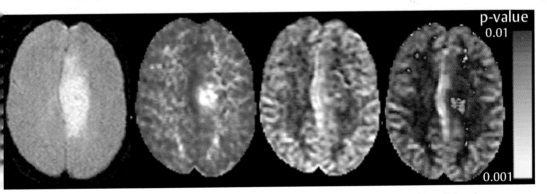

Fig. 26 Increased flow heterogeneity in angiogenic tumor. In this figure the color scale is reversed to show areas where the heterogeneity is increased compared to normal. This is a 40-year-old woman with a grade II astrocytoma.

The p value represents the likelihood that the flow heterogeneity is no different than the mean overall heterogeneity (figure courtesy of J. Rabinov and L. Østergaard).

Average vessel diameter

In Fig. 14 (p. 34) above we pointed out that for a given dose of Gd, signal change differs with vessel size particularly with SE EPI techniques. Dennie and others have proposed [33a] that one might use this difference to interrogate average capillary diameter in a voxel. This approach consists of interleaving GE and SE acquisitions during a single bolus injection of contrast. Fig. 14 above shows that as vessel size increases, $\Delta R2$ increases and peaks for vessels in the order of $1 - 2$ μm, while $\Delta R2^*$ increases, then plateaus to remain largely independent of vessel size beyond $3 - 4$ μm. However, both $\Delta R2^*$ and $\Delta R2$ depend upon the fraction of vessels in tissue as well as the $\Delta\chi$ (or change in susceptibility) which are not usually known *a priori*. One method of minimizing the dependence on these poorly defined parameters is to take the ratio of $\Delta R2^*$ to $\Delta R2$, since both $\Delta R2$ and $\Delta R2^*$ show a similar, nearly linear response to $\Delta\chi$ and vessel fraction [14]. The ratio $\Delta R2^*/\Delta R2$ increases nearly linearly with vessel size and therefore may provide an indication of the average vessel size present within a voxel which may differentiate between normal tissue and tumors. An example of this is shown in Fig. 27. While this technique remains to be fully explored, it potentially could allow for more complete characterization of microvascular anatomy.

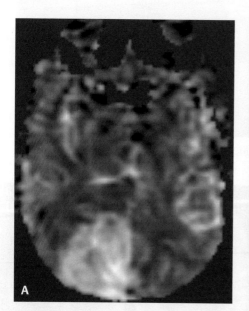 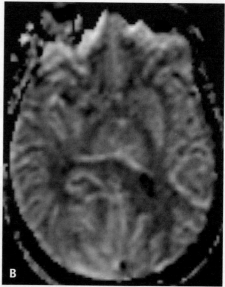

Fig. 27   Possible vessel size difference in a malignant meningioma.

(A) CBV map with gradient echo technique.
(B) CBV map with spin echo technique. Note the difference in the tumor compared to gray matter, especially in the GE image versus the SE image. The ratio of $\Delta R2^*/\Delta R2$ in the gray matter is 1.01 but 3.51 in the tumor, suggesting that the average microvessel size is much larger in the tumor.

Part 2: Perfusion Imaging in Clinical Practice

Perfusion MRI compared to other routine modalities

Perfusion MRI offers some distinct advantages to other perfusion modalities such as PET, SPECT, or X-ray CT-based methods:
- Signal to noise. The SNR and CNR of MRI perfusion is superior to other routine modalities.
- Availability. MRI is more available than PET or xenon-inhalation CT.
- Resolution. MRI has higher spatial resolution than SPECT, PET, or xenon-CT.
- Safety. MRI does not expose subjects to any form of ionizing radiation.
- Speed. Perfusion MRI can be done quickly; it can be a very minimal extension of an already-scheduled MRI exam.
- Coverage. Iodine-based CT-perfusion techniques are limited to a one or at most a few slices. Perfusion MRI, on the other hand, can easily obtain 10 slices, and more at lower resolutions.

Finally, perhaps a unique feature of MR perfusion is the sensitivity to the small vessels. Since most neuropathology occurs with some microvascular correlates, imaging of the capillaries is of particular interest. MRI can focus on these small vessels and thereby highlight pathology occurring at the capillary level. A typical series of microvascular rCBV maps in normal subjects are shown in Fig. **8** (p. 23). These can be compared to a typical positron-emission study of blood volume, Fig. **28**, which is dominated by the large vascular structures. Typical features of a normal spin echo rCBV map include a normally slightly higher rCBV in the visual cortex, and zero rCBV in the ventricles. Furthermore, note that larger vascular structures, notably cortical veins and arteries, also contribute to image contrast on these MRI CBV maps, though much less so than on the PET map.

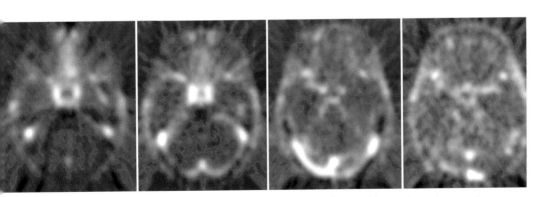

Fig. **28**   Normal CO-PET study. Note that the image is dominated by the structures with highest blood volume; in particular, the venous sinuses, with 100% blood volume, have such a high signal that gray-white differences are obscured.

Perfusion MRI in cerebrovascular disease

Acute stroke

Stroke is diagnosed in approximately 600,000 patients per year in the United States and contributes to at least 150,000 deaths per year in the US [34]. In addition to the difficulty of making an accurate diagnosis clinically (false positive rates for stroke diagnosis range up to 40%), decisions about intervention may depend on a more accurate assessment than clinical evaluation. While there is now an approved therapy for acute human stroke, thrombolysis with recombinant tissue plasminogen activator (rt-PA), many stroke sufferers do not benefit from such treatment, and indeed some are harmed by thrombolysis. Many investigators believe that the suboptimal success in treating stroke is due to an incomplete understanding of human stroke, particularly in the acute stage. It may be that imaging can provide both insight into the underlying pathophysiology of acute stroke as well as aid in the acute management of patients.

Stroke pathophysiology and imaging of blood flow

Conventional T2-weighted images and CT studies are typically abnormal 12 to 24 hours after the onset of ischemia; this is often too late to allow useful intervention, and does not allow study of the early events in cerebral ischemia. Functional MRI techniques, however, particularly perfusion MRI and diffusion MRI, have been shown to be sensitive to acute stroke in its earliest stages [35-38]. The role of perfusion MRI in the evaluation of acute stroke is best understood when placed in context with what is currently understood about cerebral hemodynamics and ischemia. Brain cells use oxygen and glucose as metabolic substrates. When either substrate is unavailable, as with acute occlusion of a major cerebral artery, metabolism is affected; if ischemia is prolonged cell death occurs. A great deal of effort has been extended in order to elucidate the pathophysiology of stroke. Although key steps remain poorly understood, it appears that the first result of ischemia is an alteration of the cellular metabolism from an aerobic to an anaerobic state. This produces increased intracellular lactate with a concomitant decrease in intracellular ATP. This decrease in the energy stores of the cell leads to a disrupted local homeostasis. This in turn can lead to a number of physiological changes, including decreased pH, increased extracellular potassium, and/or increased extracellular neurotransmitters (e.g., glutamate). This loss of homeostasis results in neuronal dysfunction, possibly with abnormal stimulation such as spreading depression and excitotoxic activity. This neuronal dysfunction (including possibly hyperstimulation) may lead to a further loss of homeostasis, particularly increased permeability of the cell membrane to calcium, in a sort of vicious circle. This hyperactivity and/or loss of homeostasis is followed by cell death. Concomitant with the cellular dysfunction is a loss of the autoregulatory function of the brain capillary bed, such that at certain stages of ischemia, reperfusion may actually increase injury rather than reverse the cellular decline [39–42].

What is the relationship between cerebral blood flow and this pathophysiological chain of events? While a complete absence of blood flow will start this chain, more typically the degree of blood flow drop is not complete. The relationship between the level of cerebral blood flow and neuronal dysfunction has been studied, and it appears that there is a level of cerebral blood flow (typically 20–30 mL/100 g/min) at which neurons stop functioning (producing observable clinical symptoms) but have not undergone cell death. Therefore, the cellular dysfunction and damage from ischemia may be reversible. This has led to the concept of an "ischemic penumbra" [43]. This penumbra has been extensively investigated in animal studies (e.g., [44]), and also in humans by means of nuclear medicine as well as MRI techniques, and currently is thought of as composed of brain tissue which is viable but ischemic. Cells in the penumbra are presumably somewhere along the series of steps described above in the pathophysiology of stroke, but may be salvageable by intervention. Importantly, the penumbra may be as much defined by the duration of the ischemic insult as by its degree of severity. A decrease in blood flow which does not produce cellular dysfunction acutely may do so if maintained for longer periods of time [47]. Furthermore, an ischemic insult which causes no discernible injury may cause infarction if it is repeated [48]. This implies that a method of visualizing not just the level of blood flow but also the degree of metabolic response to that blood flow would be of interest.

One of the goals of fMRI is to visualize the ischemic penumbra, and ideally identify at an early time point the difference between salvageable, non-salvageable, and undamaged tissue. Imaging of acute stroke has been undertaken with a variety of MRI techniques, including spectroscopic, diffusion, perfusion, and conventional imaging, all with an aim to visualize one or more of the steps in the pathophysiological process of stroke. Currently, many investigators hypothesize that the diffusion abnormality represents the tissue that has responded to the metabolic insult of stroke, whereas abnormalities on perfusion MRI that are not yet diffusion-abnormal may represent tissue at risk.

Practical perfusion MRI in acute stroke

All three of the main descriptors of perfusion (CBV, CBF, and MTT) are useful in imaging acute cerebral ischemia. Of these three, CBV maps have been shown to correlate best with final infarct volume, as shown in Fig. **29**, implying that rCBV maps may include flow that comes in via collateral vessels, and thus give a snapshot of cerebrovascular reserve. MTT is an easy-to-interpret format that is homogeneous in normal areas. This is useful because the gray-white differences that are present in CBF and CBV maps can make interpretation difficult. MTT does have a tendency to overestimate infarct size, and generally MTT maps tend towards a binary classification; they tend to show either areas as normal or else uniformly abnormal (with no gradation). This can be helpful for identifying areas of abnormal hemodynamics. Unfortunately, MTT and other timing maps do not appear to do an adequate task in distinguishing between levels of hemodynamic compromise. That is, the feature that makes them easy to interpret – being somewhat all or nothing, normal or abnormal – does not allow for the gradation of abnormalities, the difference between blood flow decreases that are mild to moderate versus moderate to severe. And of course, all of these perfusion techniques (both MRI and non-MRI) appear to be unable to distinguish between acute and chronic hemodynamic compromise. Fortunately, DWI can easily make this distinction.

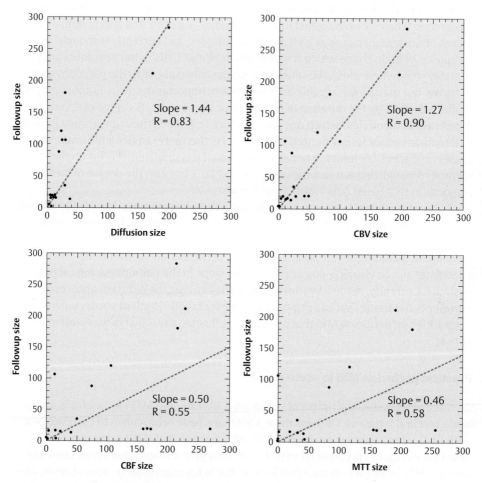

Fig. 29   Scatter plots of initial lesion volume compared to follow-up infarct volume. These demonstrate that CBV has the highest correlation to a linear fit and the slope closest to 1.0 (from Sorensen AG, Copen W, Østergaard L et al. 1999 [8]).

In routine clinical practice, we acquire DWI and a single PWI data set, and then process these data into a series of physiological images. Fig. **30** illustrates an example of DWI and PWI demonstrating acute cerebral ischemia (see also Movie Clip ⊙ **15**). Note that the DWI abnormality in this case, as in many cases, is smaller than the PWI abnormality. In some cases, the PWI abnormality is present even though the DWI is not yet abnormal. An example of this is shown in Fig. **31** (see also Movie Clips ⊙ **16** and **17**). In this example, it is noteworthy that there are two lesions present. In one there is a "penumbra" of PWI abnormality around the DWI lesion, and this area goes on to infarction. However, there is also an area of PWI abnormality that is not yet abnormal on DWI, and this too proceeds to infarction.

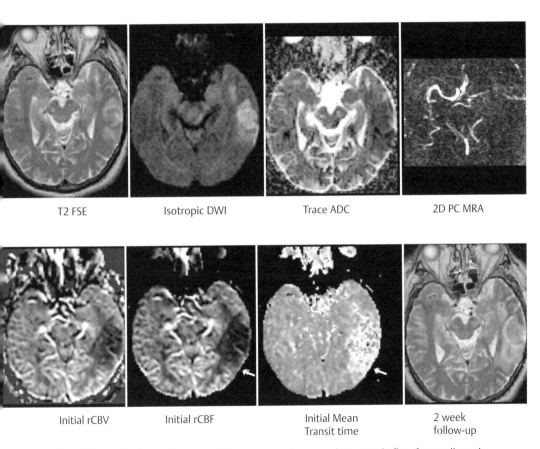

| T2 FSE | Isotropic DWI | Trace ADC | 2D PC MRA |

| Initial rCBV | Initial rCBF | Initial Mean Transit time | 2 week follow-up |

Fig. **30** Diffusion/Perfusion Mismatch. This 62-year-old male was imaged 7 hours after the sudden onset of dense right hemiplegia. T2 FSE images demonstrate minimal T2 change with slight sulcal effacement. DWI and ADC show a large area of abnormality in the left temporal lobe; the etiology of this is confirmed by the phase contrast MRA that documents left ICA occlusion and retrograde flow from collaterals. The initial rCBV, rCBF, and MTT images show the lesion, and the arrowhead point out an area posterior to the DWI abnormality that is perfusion abnormal but diffusion normal. Follow-up imaging demonstrates that this area proceeds to infarction.

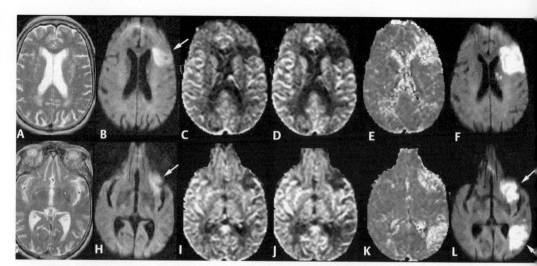

Fig. **31**   Mismatch between diffusion and perfusion. Sensitivity of rCBF and MTT to ischemia. A 78-year-old female imaged three hours after the onset of aphasia during cardiac catheterization.

(**A**) T2 weighted image is normal.
(**B**) DWI demonstrates hyperintensity in the left frontal lobe consistent with the patient's symptoms (arrow). Hemodynamic images including rCBV (**C**), rCBF (**D**), and MTT (**E**) document a similar abnormality, albeit slightly larger.
(**F**) Follow-up diffusion-weighted image at 5 days documents infarction.
(**G**) T2 image again shows no abnormality on a lower slice.

(**H**) DWI documents an inferior frontal lobe hyperintensity consistent with ischemia (arrow), but no hyperintensity in the left occipital lobe. Hemodynamic imaging shows both the DWI abnormal area, and a new area of threatened tissue in the occipital region. This is not seen on rCBV (**I**), but is shown on the other two images as a 75% drop in rCBF (**J**) and a doubling of MTT. (**K**) Follow-up imaging confirms the second area of infarct as well as the first (arrows) (**L**) (figure from Sorensen AG, Copen W, Østergaard L et al. 1999 [8]). See Movie Clips ⊙ **16** and **17**.

This DWI/PWI mismatch has been considered as a possible imaging correlate to the ischemic penumbra. It can be instructive to note how the various PWI images depict these regions, and the insight that they can bring. Fig. **32** demonstrates how MTT and CBF maps can overestimate eventual infarct while CBV and DWI tend to be more closely correlated (see also Movie Clip ⊙ **18**). This is simply an example of the tendencies shown in Figs. **29** above, where CBV and DWI have the highest correlation but CBF and MTT tend to overestimate. This tendency is probably due to the ability of the brain to withstand some decreased CBF but compensate somehow, either through autoregulatory mechanisms or via collateral flow. Some groups now have documented that the perfusion can play a helpful role in defining tissue at risk [42, 49–53] and clinical outcome [54–56].

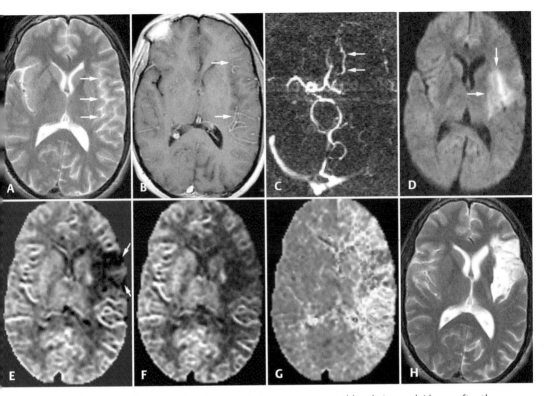

Fig. 32 Specificity of rCBV, rCBF, and MTT to ischemia. A 33-year-old male imaged 4 hours after the onset of right sided hemiplegia and mutism.

(**A**) T2 weighted image shows sulcal effacement (arrows).
(**B**) Post-contrast T1-weighted images demonstrate contrast in multiple dilated vessels in the affected hemisphere, consistent with slow flow (arrows).
(**C**) Phase-contrast MRA demonstrates absence of flow in the left ICA and MCA. Note the prominent ophthalmic artery (arrows), which directional MRA demonstrated had retrograde flow (not shown).
(From Sorensen AG, Copen W, Østergaard L et al. 1999 [8]). See Movie Clip ⊙ **18**.

(**D**) DWI demonstrates hyperintensity in the left hemisphere consistent with the patient's symptoms (arrows).
Hemodynamic images including rCBV (**E**), rCBF (**F**), and MTT (**G**) document a larger area of blood flow decrease than blood volume (arrows) or DWI abnormality, consistent with the MCA branch occlusion but with collateral flow.
(**H**) Follow-up T2-weighted image at 7 months documents the infarction is smaller than the flow abnormality but larger than the diffusion abnormality.

In our experience, the overestimation by MTT seems to be more severe when gradient echo EPI is used rather than SE EPI. Fig. **33** shows this well, with a large area abnormal by MTT but demonstrating on CBF only a moderate drop, with only punctate areas going on to infarction. The ability to get even relative CBF values can greatly increase the diagnostic specificity of an exam. This can help distinguish between a lesion that needs acute treatment versus a lesion that may be chronic.

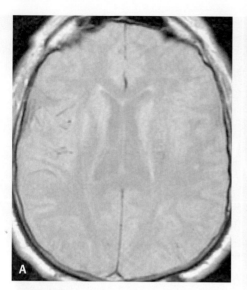
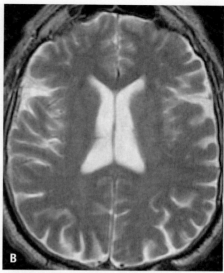

Fig. 33   Diffusion and perfusion abnormalities in a 55-year-old male 2 hours after the onset of right hemiparesis.

(A) and (B) Proton-density-weighted and T2-weighted FSE images, respectively, demonstrate no abnormality.

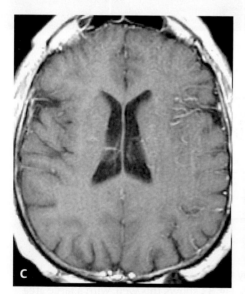
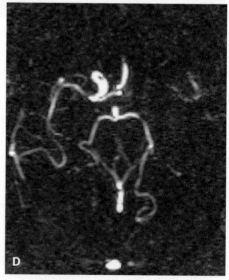

(C) Post-contrast T1-weighted images demonstrate intravascular enhancement.

(D) 2 D PC MRA demonstrates absence of flow in the left ICA and proximal MCA, but some retrograde filling of the distal MCA.

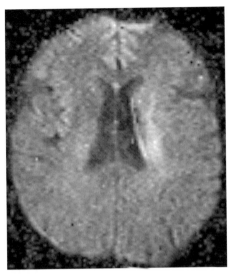

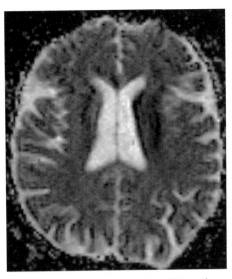

33 (**E**) DWI demonstrates a small area of hyperintense signal in the periventricular white matter.

33 (**F**) This same area has a low ADC on the trace ADC maps, confirming the ischemic event

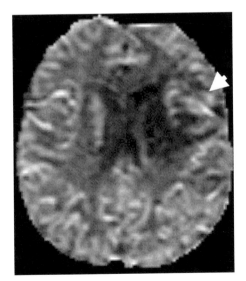

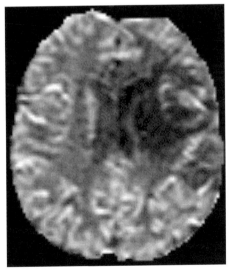

33 (**G**) A much larger rCBV abnormality is evident, though there are areas with high rCBV around the diffusion abnormality (arrowhead).

33 (**H**) A core of decreased rCBF is evident.

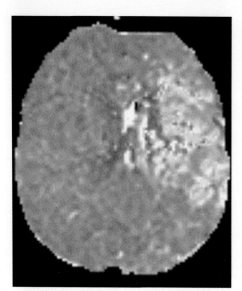

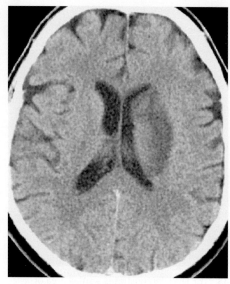

33   (**I**) A large MTT abnormality is present.

33   (**J**) Follow-up CT after 3 days of hypertensive therapy demonstrates a lesion larger than the DWI abnormality but smaller than the rCBV map abnormality, implying the tissue at risk as demonstrated by intravascular enhancement (**C**) and rCBV abnormality (**G**) benefited from the hypertensive therapy. (In part from Sorensen AG, Copen W, Østergaard L et al. 1999 [8].)

One important thing to remember about rCBV, particularly in the setting of acute cerebral ischemia, is that the way CBV maps are made typically leaves them with some CBF-weighting. Consider the difference between an animal study of severe ischemia where a CBV contrast agent might be injected before the ischemic event, and a human study of severe ischemia where the contrast agent is injected only after the event. In both cases, it is thought that vasodilatation occurs as the vascular bed attempts to drop intravascular pressure to increase flow. In the animal case, it is quite likely that the measured CBV would increase, because there would be contrast agent available to pool in the dilated capillaries. However, in the human, if the ischemic insult is severe enough, the contrast agent may not be able to reach the area of increased CBV, because the vessel that would feed that area of the brain is occluded. On the other hand, it appears that in areas where the contrast can reach, in the peri-infarct zone, often CBV is elevated as predicted. An example of this is shown in Fig. **32** (see also Movie Clip ⊙ **18**); in a study of 23 subjects, Sorensen et al. found such elevations in 8 subjects[8]. Other studies have confirmed that CBV can be elevated or decreased depending on the level of hypoperfusion[42,57]. Furthermore, rCBV can be elevated in some non-acute pathiophysiological states; one study reported that white matter rCBV was elevated in unilateral internal carotid artery occlusion[58].

Reperfusion

The brain's response to acute cerebral ischemia is to activate mechanisms to lyse the clot. In approximately 20% of cases studied with angiography, spontaneous thrombolysis occurs in the first 24 hours[59]. Perfusion MRI can play a particularly valuable role in identifying reperfusion, since the DWI and T2 images may still be either normal or abnormal in such regions. Identification of reperfusion is important for two therapeutic reasons. First, if reperfusion has occurred, then thrombolytic therapy should be avoided. Second, other types of therapy, such as hypertensive therapy, might also be contraindicated, since once reperfusion has occurred there appears to be an increased risk of hemorrhagic transformation. Figs. **34** and **35** demonstrate examples of reperfusion highlighted by perfusion MRI. Note that often the area of reperfusion does not have normal blood flow or blood volume, but actually shows increased CBF and/or CBV. The increase in CBF without a concomitant increase in metabolic demand is termed "luxury perfusion". Reperfusion is also thought to be associated with additional injury to the brain; so-called reperfusion injury is the target of a number of neuroprotective strategies.

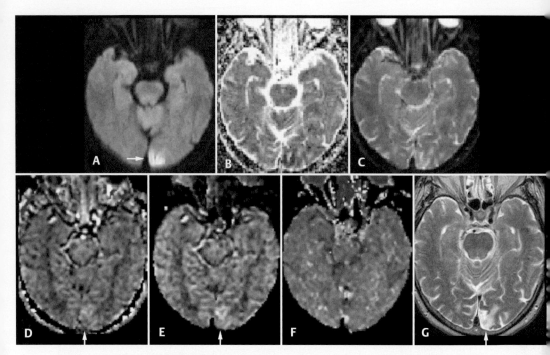

Fig. 34   Spontaneous reperfusion. A 69-year-old male imaged 10 hours after the onset of a right quadrantanopia and left-sided numbness.

Diffusion-weighted imaging (**A**) and trace ADC maps (**B**) document abnormal water mobility in the left occipital lobe (arrow).
Echo-planar T2-weighted imaging (**C**) was also subtly abnormal (conventional T2 images were degraded by a motion artifact).
Hemodynamic imaging including rCBV (**D**), rCBF (**E**), and MTT (**F**) document increased blood flow and blood volume (arrows) in the area of diffusion abnormality, suggesting spontaneous reperfusion.

Follow-up at 9 months (**G**) showed infarction (arrow) with focal low rCBV (not shown). The ability to document such spontaneous reperfusion may help identify patients no longer in need of chemical or mechanical thrombolysis. Such patients can thereby avoid the risks associated with thrombolytic therapy (from Sorensen AG, Copen W, Østergaard L et al. 1999 [8]). See also Movie Clip ⊙ **19.**

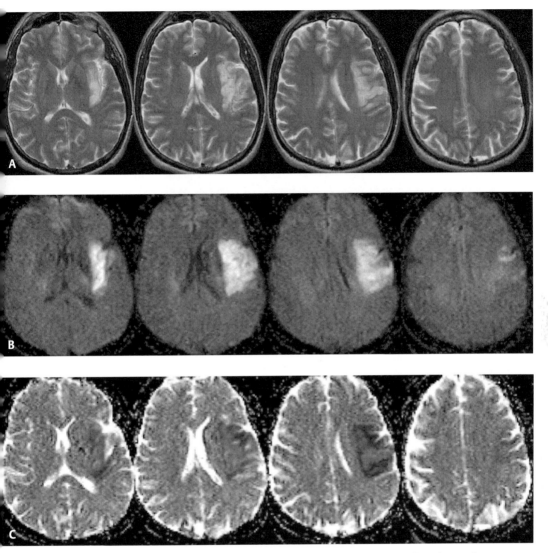

Fig. 35 Reperfusion in subacute setting. A 51-year-old male imaged approximately 36 hours after left carotid endarterectomy and symptoms of acute intra-operative ischemic stroke. Angiography at approximately 12 hours post operation demonstrated occlusion of a superior branch of the left MCA.

This MRI study now shows infarction on T2 images (**A**), DWI (**B**), and ADC maps (**C**), all consistent with recent infarction.

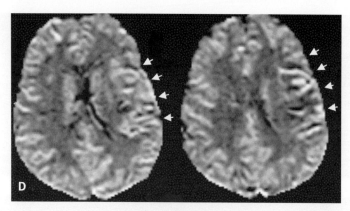

35   Of note, CBV (**D**), CBF (**E**), and MTT (**F**) images all demonstrate hyperemia, with elevated CBV, elevated CBF, and decreased MTT. See also Movie Clip ⊙ **20**.

rCBV elevated 26 %

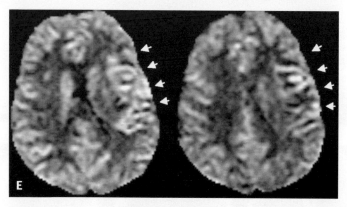

rCBV elevated 55 %

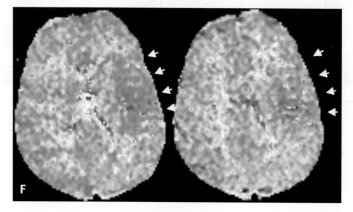

MTT decreased 19 %

Chronic stroke

While assessment of acute stroke has clear clinical utility, perfusion MRI may also be useful in the management of chronic stroke. Approximately one-sixth to one-quarter of stroke patients hospitalized annually for stroke have recurrent disease [60,61]. Assessment of patient pathology after stroke may help identify patients who may benefit from intervention. For example, delay in the time to peak signal change after a bolus of contrast agent has been correlated with the degree of carotid artery stenosis in humans [62]. However, one must be careful to distinguish mere delay due to stenosis, as is common, from actual decreased CBF that might indicate a risk for near-term infarction. Fig. **36** demonstrates how MTT calculated using the *contralateral* (and normal) MCA can highlight a large abnormality. However, both Figs. **36** and **37** demonstrate how such areas of abnormal arrival time may in fact often turn out to be overestimates if the wrong AIF is chosen. It is important to recognize the difference between timing differences, which may not be meaningful and can be accounted for by examining the AIF, and true flow decreases. Fig. **38** indicates perfusion maps in a patient with an extracranial-to-intracranial bypass graft; in this case some of the timing differences could be attributed solely to the longer time it takes the blood to go up the external carotid, through the skull, and into the brain.

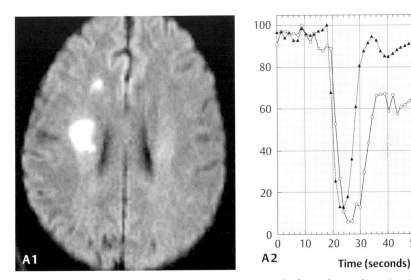

Fig. **36**   Perfusion study in a 39-year-old female one month after right ICA dissection. Her diffusion-weighted image showed ongoing ischemia. Her perfusion maps show defects that vary considerably when the right MCA is used as the arterial input function versus the left MCA.

(**A1**) DWI showing deep ischemia.

(**A2**) Graphs of the signal intensity (arbitrary values) versus time show that the R MCA AIF is delayed and broader compared to the L MCA AIF.

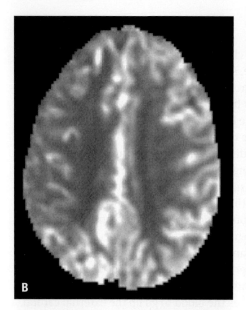

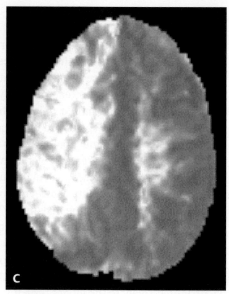

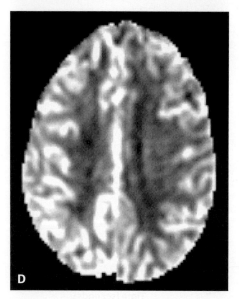

36   (**B–D**) CBF, MTT, and CBV maps respectively using the left MCA as an arterial input function show a large defect in flow in the right hemisphere.

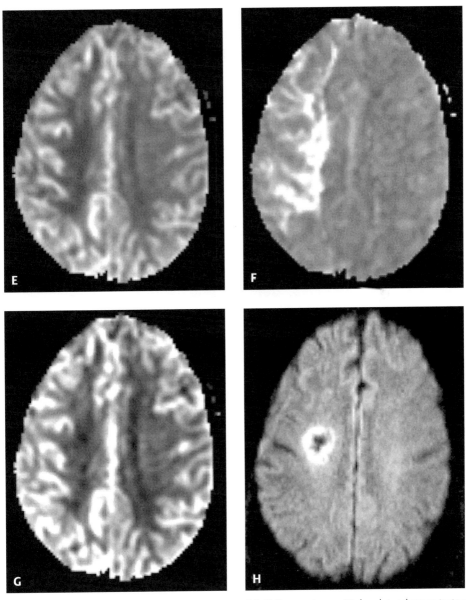

36 (**E–G**) CBF, MTT, and CBV maps using the right MCA as the AIF show a much smaller defect.

(**H**) Follow-up image 10 days later demonstrates that the infarct has not grown and that the majority of the transit time abnormality was due to delay.

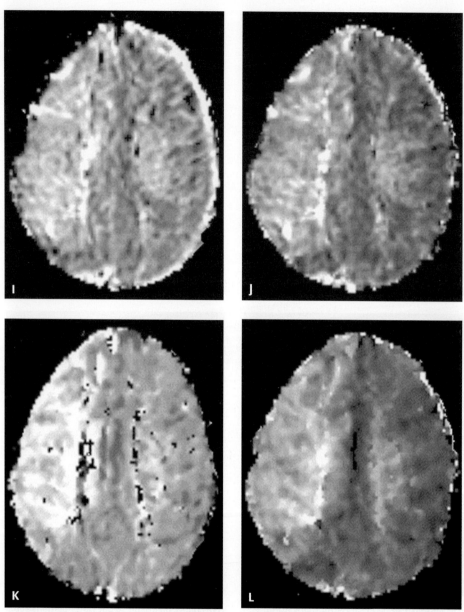

36 Other hemodynamic maps such as area over peak (**I**), full width half max (**J**), arrival time (**K**), and time to peak (**L**) all are subject to these delay issues. Compare the size of the lesion on the hemodynamic maps that use no AIF (maps **I–L**) or an inappropriate AIF (maps **B–D**) to those that use an appropriate AIF (maps **E–G**). See also Movie Clip ⊙ **21.**

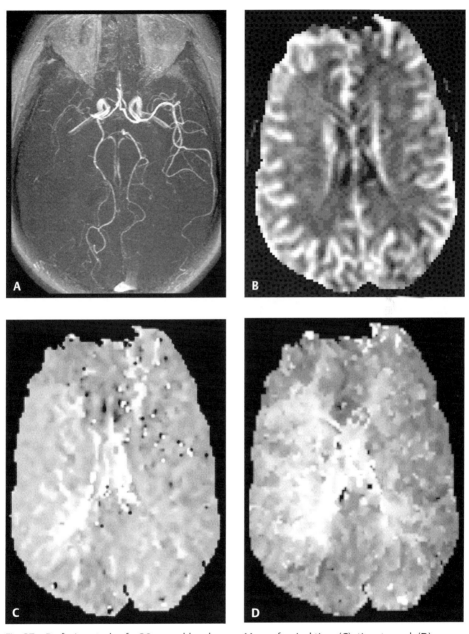

Fig. 37   Perfusion study of a 26-year-old male with long-standing right MCA narrowing seen on MRA (**A**).
The total CBV is normal (**B**), indicating that the brain tissue is being perfused well, possibly by collaterals.

Maps of arrival time (**C**), time to peak (**D**), or mean transit time using the left MCA (the normal MCA).

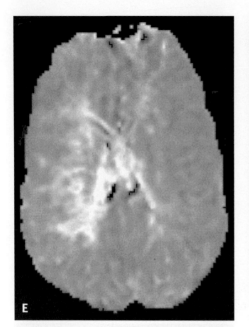

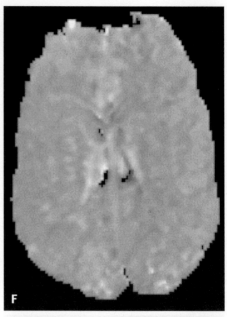

37   (**E**) as the AIF all highlight large abnormalities. However, the MTT abnormality is essentially nonexistent when the right MCA is used as the arterial input function (**F**). This study was done at 3.0 T on a General Electric Signa system modified for EPI by Advanced NMR. See also Movie Clip ⊙ **22**.

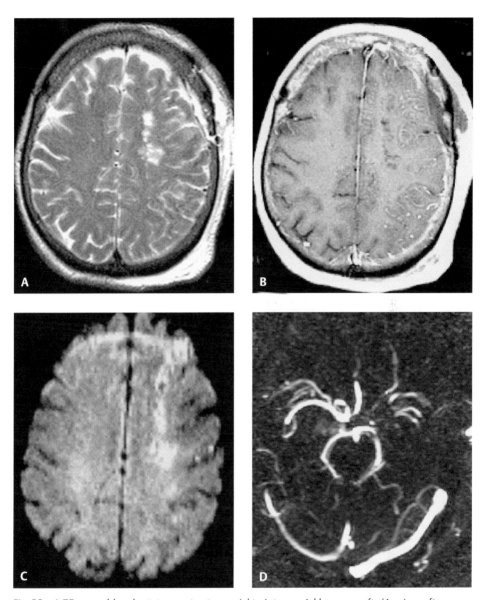

Fig. 38   A 75-year-old male status post extracranial to intracranial bypass graft. (A vein graft was used to connect the common carotid artery to an opercular branch of the middle cerebral artery.)

T2-weighted images (**A**), T1 post-contrast images (**B**), and diffusion-weighted images (**C**) all show evidence of deep ischemia with some cortical vascular enhancement suggesting slow cortical flow.

The 2 D phase contrast MRA (**D**) demonstrates the graft is patent but the left ICA is not. Perfusion studies indicate that both regional hyperperfusion and hypoperfusion is present.

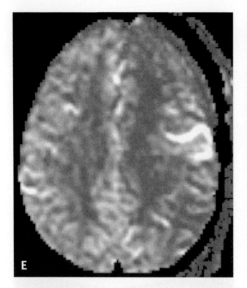

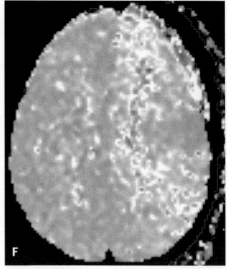

38   This is visualized on maps of CBF (**E**), MTT (**F**), and CBV (**G**). Note the areas of shortened (dark) MTT in the center of the right hemisphere, surrounded by longer (brighter) MTT indicating hyperperfusion surrounded by hypoperfusion. See also Movie Clip ⊙ **23**.

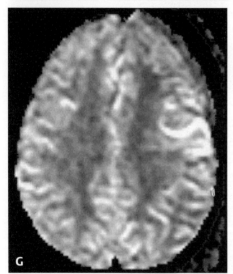

Moya-moya

Chronic large vessel obstruction leads to the puff-of-smoke angiographic appearance termed moya-moya. This abnormality, like vasospasm, is a diffuse one. The MCA or other large vessel, even if it could be found, would probably not be the proper AIF for many of the voxels in the brain. Nevertheless, there are still many detectable abnormalities in hemodynamics [63,64]; the question instead becomes what is the likelihood of such abnormalities representing a lesion that needs to be treated. This is usually best determined by obtaining a baseline scan and then comparing subsequent imaging sessions to the initial scan. Fig. **39** shows an example of perfusion imaging in a patient with proven moya-moya disease. The dynamic images in such a subject can be particularly helpful.

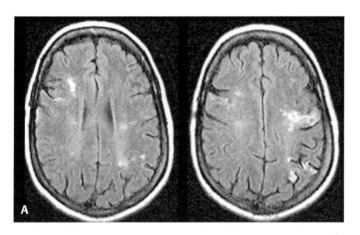

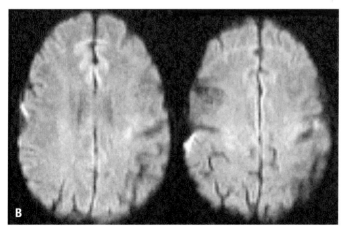

Fig. **39**   A 36-year-old patient with moya-moya.

FLAIR images (**A**) and diffusion-weighted images (**B**) highlight the chronic changes present. Note the differing patterns of perfusion abnormalities based on the arterial input function chosen. For each triplet, the left MCA, the right PCA, and the right MCA are chosen, respectively.

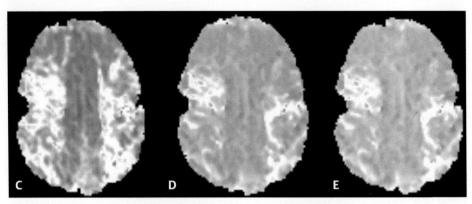

39   (**C – E**) MTT.

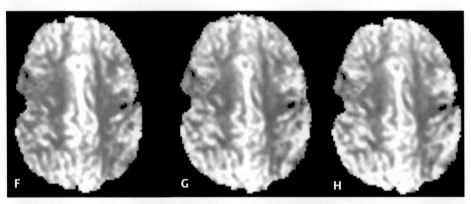

39   (**F – H**): CBF.

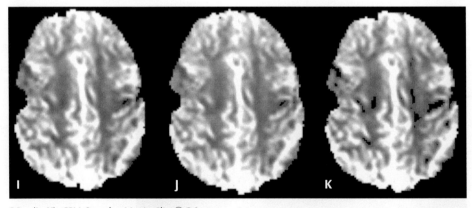

39   (**I – K**) CBV. See also Movie Clip ⊙ **24**.

Intraparenchymal hemorrhage

While the imaging of intraparenchymal hemorrhage is trivial with MRI, since MRI is so sensitive to very small mass lesions within the brain, the effects of the hemorrhage may be more difficult to detect. Perfusion MRI can be sensitive to the changes in blood flow around a hemorrhage. This is despite the susceptibility effects from a hematoma. Again, use of SE EPI techniques can help in this regard since the SE technique will refocus some of the signal loss. Fig. **40** demonstrates perfusion MRI in a case of probable amyloid angiopathy with intracranial hemorrhage.

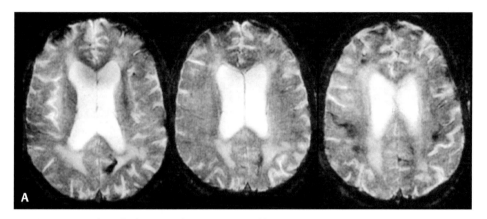

Fig. **40**   Presumed amyloid angiopathy in a 76-year-old man.

Gradient echo images (**A**) demonstrate multiple areas of decreased signal consistent with hemosiderin deposition.

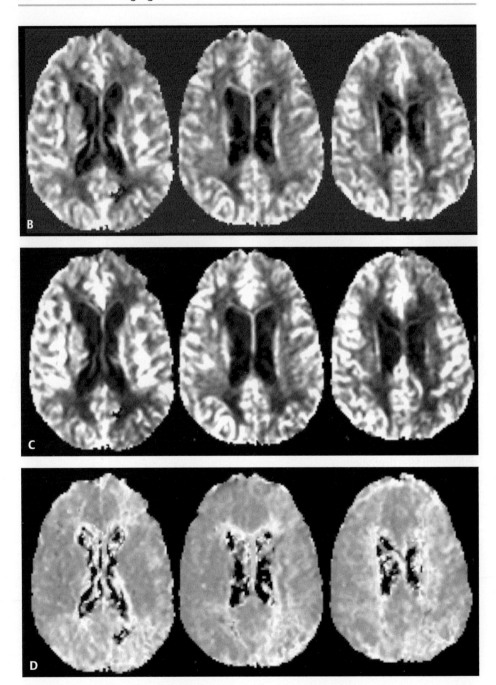

40   Maps of CBV (**B**), CBF (**C**), and MTT
(**D**) demonstrate regional areas of decreased
flow change consistent with old white matter
ischemic change and cortical atrophy. Note that
the hemosiderin causes signal loss on the computed images as well; this is even more apparent
on the raw image data, see Movie Clip ⊙ **25**.

Intracranial tumors

Rationale for perfusion MRI[139]

Diagnosis of the presence of CNS tumors has been greatly aided by MRI and its outstanding anatomic detail. Characterization of a tumor's malignant potential can be more difficult using conventional techniques, particularly because T1 and T2 relaxation times as well as the integrity of the blood-brain barrier of neoplastic tissue are only moderately specific indicators of malignancy[65–67]. Over the last several years a variety of other parameters has been sought that might be imaged *in vivo* and improve tumor characterization. These include measures of tumor growth rate, metabolism, angiogenesis, and, with MR spectroscopy, tissue chemical signatures. Much of the metabolic marker imaging has been done with nuclear technologies, especially PET and SPECT. For example, positron emission tomography studies of tumor metabolism using [18]FDG have shown the degree of glucose utilization to be a predictor of prognosis[68,69], though again this predictive value is in groups of lesions, with only moderate predictive value. Indeed, the sensitivity and specificity of PET and SPECT have been called into question by a number of investigators[70,71].

Recently, there has been interest in tumor angiogenesis. In order to continue growth, a new tumor must induce new capillary vessels once it reaches a few millimeters in size; this is termed angiogenesis. In 1991, Weidner et al.[72] demonstrated that in breast carcinoma the number of capillaries per microscopic high power field correlated linearly with the risk of metastasis. Similar findings have now been described in lung, prostate[73], and brain cancer[74]. The authors ascribed this to a biphasic behavior of tumors: a prevascular phase, which may last for years, during which there is limited tumor growth; and a vascular phase, in which there is bleeding, a high rate of tumor growth, and possible metastasis. Additional investigation has demonstrated that in *in vivo* animal studies glucose and oxygen utilization in cancer cells is limited not by the metabolic demand of the cancer cells but rather by the substrate supply, that is, the capillary bed[75]. These findings imply that important imaging markers of malignancy may include direct measurement of the microvasculature.

These findings in breast and other carcinomas are relevant to understanding primary cerebral neoplasms: the degree of angiogenesis has been linked to tumor grade in human gliomas, with higher grade lesions showing increased angiogenic factors such as renin[76] or capillary growth factors[77,78]. The role of vascular proliferation in brain tumors clearly plays a major role in the degree of malignancy. For example, the histological characteristics of glioblastoma include[79]: (1) high cell density; (2) cellular pleomorphism; (3) mitoses; (4) necroses with palisading cells; and (5) prominent vascularization with endothelial cell proliferation[80,81]. In a major study of 1440 malignant astrocytic gliomas, Burger et al. noted that only vascular proliferation differentiated anaplastic astrocytomas into short- and long-term survival categories;

"no other features showed such a significant association with either short or long survival" [82]. Perfusion MRI, with its sensitivity to the capillary bed, especially when using spin echo techniques, may therefore be ideally suited for evaluating tumor angiogenesis *in vivo*. In recent years considerable clinical experience has been gained with perfusion MR imaging of tumors. Perfusion MRI can play an important role at the major clinical decision points: diagnosis, intervention, and post-treatment monitoring.

Diagnosis

Glial lesions

No systematic long-term studies of perfusion MRI in the diagnosis of brain tumors have been published, however, numerous small series have been reported. Since maps of CBF have become available only recently, most published tumor perfusion MRI work focuses on rCBV. In a study of 29 patients comparing fMRI rCBV with ^{18}FDG PET and pathological grade, good correlation was found between tumor grade on biopsy, rCBV, and FDG uptake [83,84]. This relative paucity of data suggests the comparative youth of perfusion MRI. Nevertheless, some conclusions about perfusion MRI and its role in diagnosis can be drawn.

The most common primary CNS neoplasm has historically been astrocytoma, although some believe CNS lymphoma may now be the most common [85] based on historical trends and the effects of HIV. In astrocytomas, histological tumor grade at diagnosis is the major predictor of survival [86]. Patients with grade I/IV (on the Daumas-Duport grading scale) have a median survival of 8 – 10 years, while those presenting with grade IV/IV have a median survival of 11 months [87]. Hence, high grade lesions are usually treated aggressively. Despite the fact that no well-designed, controlled trial has shown any benefit for any treatment of low grade lesions [88], in many cases treatment is offered nonetheless.

While standard radiological criteria can provide some suggestions regarding the aggressiveness of a lesion, most treatment is based upon biopsy. MRI and neuroradiologists typically play a key role in guiding tumor sampling. Destruction of the blood-brain barrier has typically been thought of as a correlative of high grade, in part because of the relationship between permeability (possibly due to increased levels of vascular endothelial growth factor, or VEGF) and angiogenesis; however, not all studies agree with this relationship [89]. In any event, finding the highest grade portion of the tumor to biopsy is important but can be challenging. For example, 25 % of lesions appear to be undergraded at stereotactic biopsy, most likely as a result of failure to sample the highest-grade portion of the lesion [90,91]. A high-resolution mapping of the grade of neoplasms that could guide biopsy would reduce this undergrading phenomenon. Perfusion maps might be able to provide such detail; candidate parameters include rCBV, flow/volume mismatches or areas of increased MTT, or possibly areas of highest BBB permeability.

Interpretation of rCBV images is typically done in a similar fashion to the interpretation of PET or other functional modalities. In PET scanning, the uptake of tracer in the region of a known lesion is typically compared with the normal gray and white matter [92]. High grades are defined as having similar or greater uptake than gray matter; often the lesions are obvious as a "hot spot" with even greater signal than gray matter [93]. A similar grading scheme has been used for rCBV mapping (at least, when using spin echo EPI). These data have indicated that tumors with any regional rCBV value (i.e., the maximum rCBV value anywhere within the tumor) over twice that of white matter (roughly comparable to gray matter) have a high likelihood of having high grade components [83] while tumors with maximum rCBV values less than 1.5 times white matter are usually low grade. Fig. **41** shows a typical low grade lesion, while Fig. **42** shows a typical high grade lesion. Often both high and low rCBV values are present in high grade lesions [94]. An important caveat here is the differentiation of a small focus of tumor neovascular proliferation from the high rCBV apparent from large vascular structures that may be adjacent to expansile lesions or the highly vascular choroid plexus If questions exist, the rCBV maps should be interpreted in concert with flow sensitive images (such as short TE gradient echoes) and the conventional post-contrast T1 weighted studies from comparable slices to avoid these potential pitfalls.

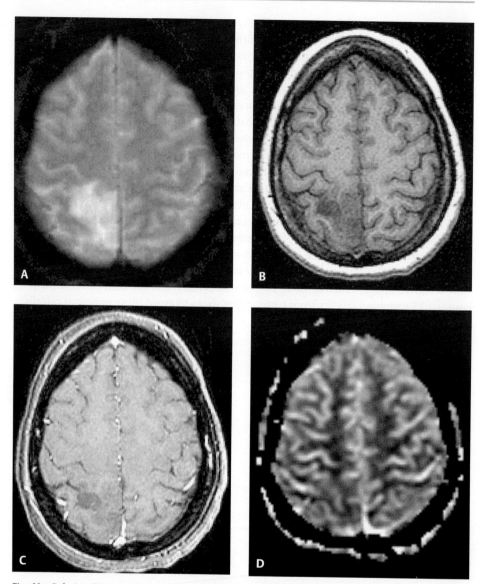

Fig. **41** Relative CBV maps in a low grade oligodendoglioma with some astrocytic components in a 39-year-old woman.

(**A**) The T2-weighted image shows lesion with minimal mass effect.
T1-weighted images pre (**B**) and post (**C**) contrast demonstrate minimal enhancement.

Map of rCBV (**D**) demonstrates a slight decrease in rCBV compared to gray matter (from Sorensen AG, Rosen B 1996 [138]).

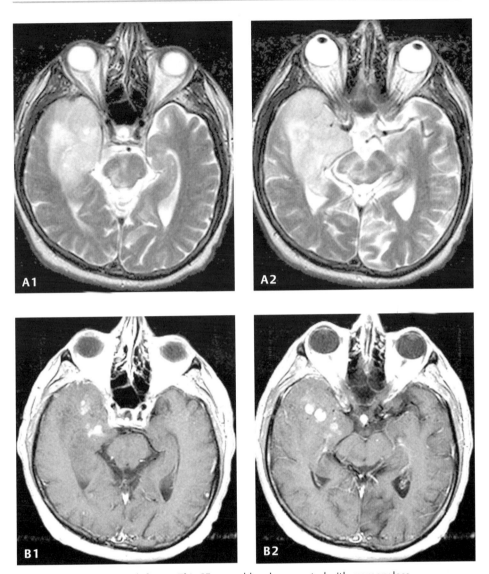

Fig. **42**   Glioblastoma multiforme. This 65-year-old male presented with memory loss, gait disturbance, and left-sided weakness.

T2-weighted images (**A 1, A 2**) and post-contrast T1-weighted images (**B 1, B 2**) demonstrate a temporal mass with variable enhancement consistent with a high grade lesion.

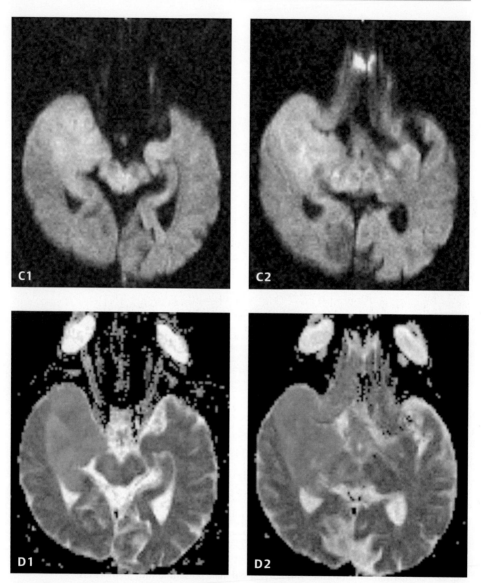

42 Diffusion-weighted imaging (**C 1, C 2**) and ADC maps (**D 1, D 2**) demonstrate mildly elevated ADC with "T2-shine through" causing mildly bright signal on the DWI images.

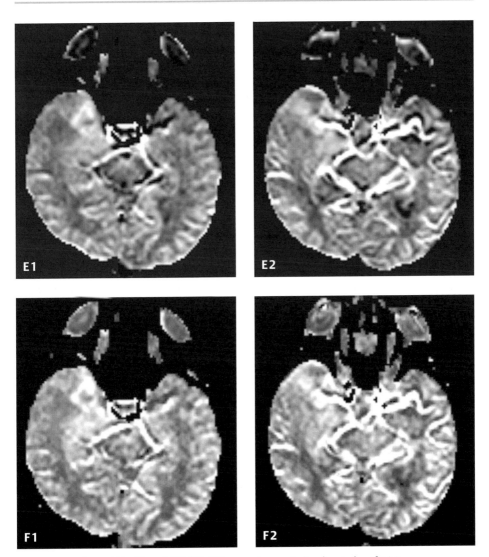

42   Corrected CBV (**E1, E2**) and CBF (**F1, F2**) maps demonstrate elevated perfusion.

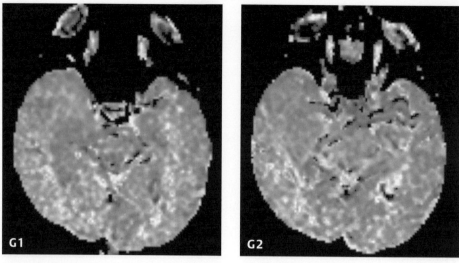

42 Note that the MTT maps (**G1,G2**) are smoothly homogeneous. Interestingly, at autopsy there were features of this lesion that favored gliomatosis cerebri. See also Movie Clips ⊙ **26** and **27**.

While rCBV does appear to indicate capillary density, it appears that oligoden-drogliomal can have an increased capillary count without a higher degree of malignancy. This higher capillary density can lead to such benign lesions having a high rCBV. Figs. **43** and **44** show an example of low grade oligodendroglial lesions mixed with more malignant glial lesions.

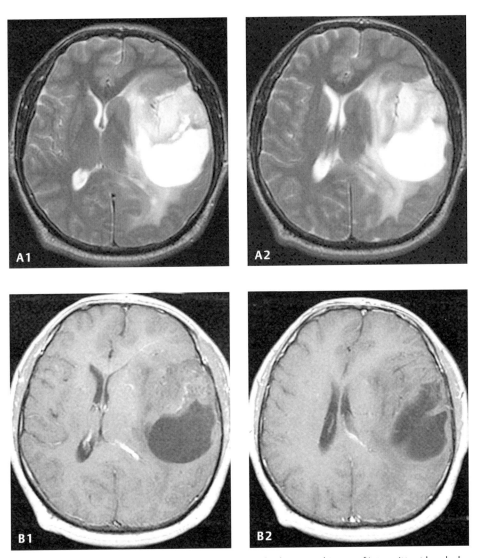

Fig. **43** Malignant mixed glioma. This 35-year-old man had a 3-year history of intermittent headache and intermittent attacks of speech arrest. Biopsy revealed mixed oligodendoglioma (about 70% of the tumor volume) and grade III glioma. Pathological examination of the high perfusion portion of the lesion demonstrated predominantly oligodendoglioma component.

T2-weighted images (**A1,A2**) and T1 post-contrast-weighted images (**B1,B2**) demonstrate that the lesion has some features of a low grade lesion, with large size but only moderate enhancement and moderate mass effect.

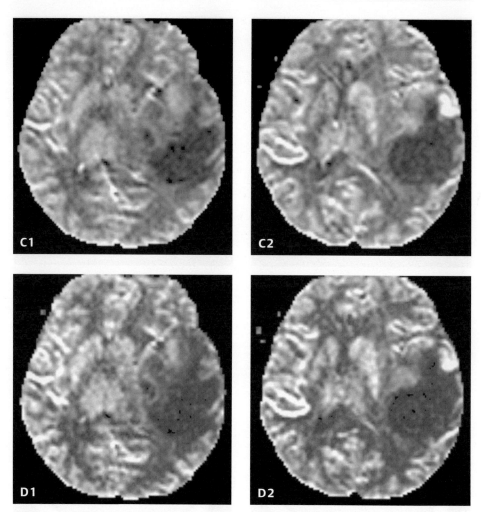

43 Maps of corrected CBV (**C1, C2**) and CBF (**D1, D2**) demonstrate some foci of high CBV and CBF but predominantly low CBV and CBF.

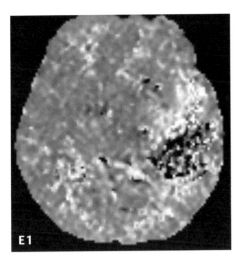 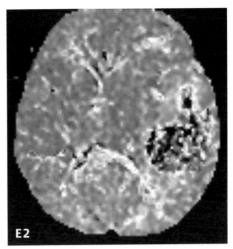

43 MTT images (**E 1, E 2**) demonstrate mis-matches in numerous areas, also consistent with low grade tumor. The completely black areas on the MTT image such as in the center of the lesion and in the center of the ventricles are where there was too little signal to create accurate maps. See also Movie Clips ⊙ **28** and **29**.

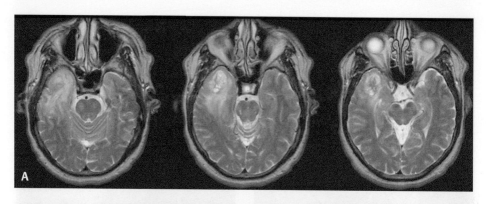

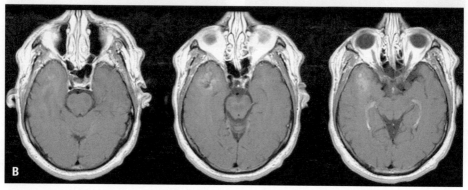

Fig. 44   Mixed oligoastrocytoma.

(A) T2-weighted images in this 49-year-old man demonstrate a right temporal lobe lesion.

(B) Post-contrast T1-weighted images demonstrate only mild to moderate enhancement.

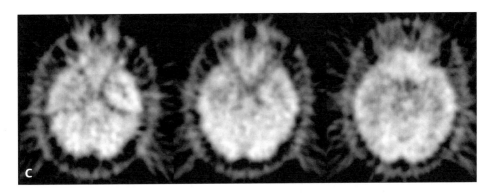

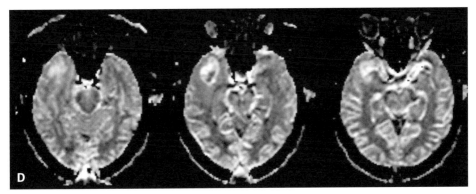

44 **(C)** Positron emission tomography images of 18 FDG demonstrate a possible high uptake focus in the center of the lesion, though prospectively was interpreted as showing no high grade lesion.

(D) Relative CBV maps demonstrate clear elevation of microvascular blood volume, suggesting numerous capillaries. Biopsy showed both an oligodendroglial component and a grade III/IV glial malignancy. Whether this high capillary count is due to the angiogenic nature of oligodendrogliomas or whether gliomas cause high CBV is an area of active investigation (from Sorensen AG, Rosen B 1996 [138]).

Preliminary studies appear to indicate that the sensitivity and specificity of rCBV is in the 70–80% range, and similar to or better than PET-FDG or SPECT [95–98]. This also appears to be the case for spin-labeling CBF approaches, though again the data are quite preliminary [99,100].

Permeability can also be assessed at the same time as rCBV, as indicated in the discussion above on BBB-breakdown correction methodology. Because the same factors that cause angiogenesis also can cause increased capillary permeability (e.g., VEGF), some investigators believe that assessment of permeability can be a valuable addition to the diagnostic armamentarium. Essentially, the correction factor that is used to correct for BBB permeability can be used directly to assess the permeability-surface area product [24,101]. This could be important if the relationship between permeability and clinical outcome is strong, as some have suggested [102].

Lymphoma

Only limited experience regarding MR perfusion imaging in lymphoma has been published at the time of this writing. One publication reports that lymphoma tends to have rCBV values lower than gray matter or hypervascular tumor but higher than white matter [103]. Another study comparing lymphoma to toxoplasmosis reported high rCBV in all six untreated active lymphomas but low rCBV in six toxoplasmosis lesions [104]. Preliminary experience at our institution also suggests that lesions with traditionally high nuclear to cytoplasm ratios have low rCBV [105]. Fig. **45** highlights an example of our experience with this lesion: its dense cellularity reflects a vascularity similar to or slightly lower than that of gray matter.

Extra-axial lesions

Because extra-axial lesions often have a relatively limited differential diagnosis and a different therapeutic approach, little perfusion MRI has been performed and no series have been published. Fig. **46** demonstrates a perfusion study in an extra-axial malignant meningioma.

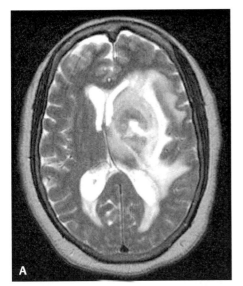

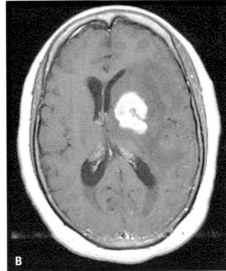

Fig. 45 Primary CNS lymphoma. A 58-year-old woman presented with three weeks of forgetfulness, right-hand clumsiness, slurred speech, and unsteady balance.

T2 images (**A**), T1-post contrast images (**B**), and FLAIR images (**C**) demonstrate an enhancing mass in the right putamen with surrounding edema. There is central necrosis and a small amount of central hemorrhage.

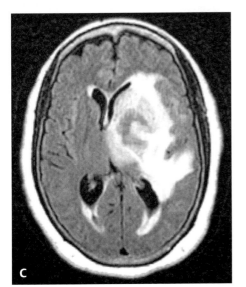

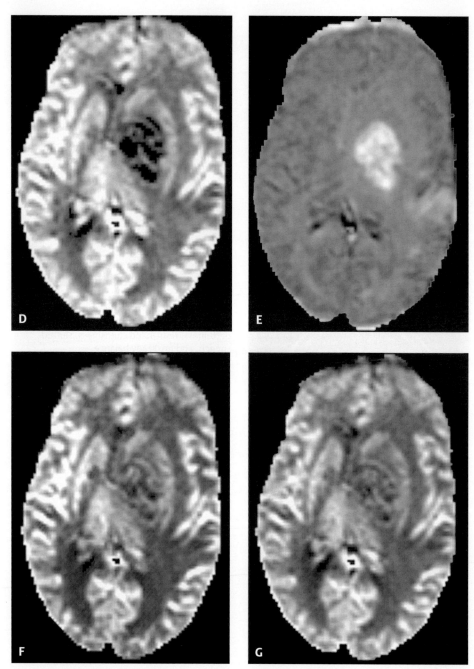

45 Perfusion images including CBV un-corrected for leakage (UCBV) (**D**), blood-brain barrier breakdown, or permeability-surface area product (sometimes colloquially referred to as K2) (**E**), CBF (**F**), and CBV corrected for BBB breakdown (cCBV) (**G**) demonstrate heterogeneous flow and volume throughout the lesion.

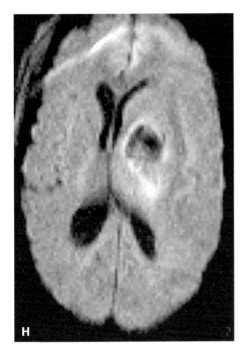

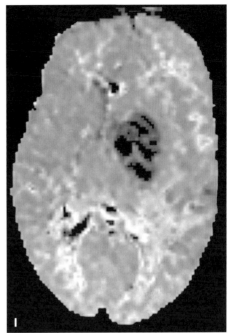

45 DWI (**H**) shows some T2 shine through in the surrounding tissues, and MTT (**I**) demonstrates insufficient SNR to make meaningful maps in the center of the lesion. Note the extensive BBB breakdown and how the corrected CBV map shows CBV within the lesion. See also Movie Clip ⊙ **30**.

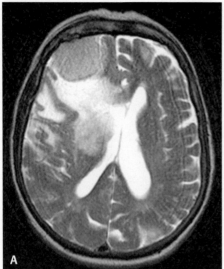

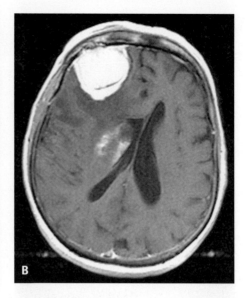

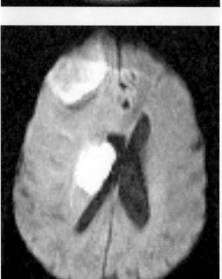

Fig. **46** Meningioma and stroke. A 90-year-old female with changes in personality was found by family members after a fall.

T2 images (**A**) and T1 post-contrast images (**B**) demonstrate both a frontal meningioma and also a mildly enhancing lesion in the right basal ganglia.
Diffusion-weighted imaging (**C**) indicates ischemia in the basal ganglia.

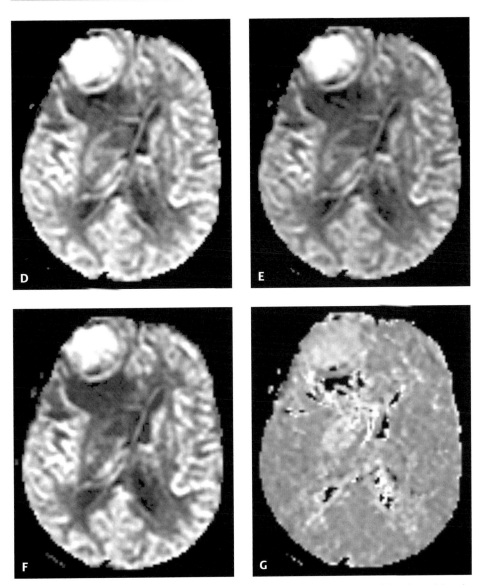

46 Perfusion imaging demonstrates high corrected CBV (**D**), uncorrected CBV (**E**) and CBF (**F**) and MTT (**G**) in the meningioma. There is low CBV and CBF and high MTT in the infarct.

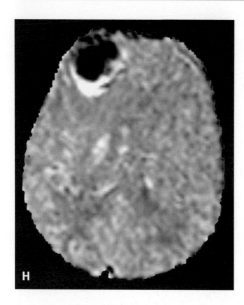

46   Note that although enhancement is evident on the T1 post-contrast image in the meningioma (**B**), the map of permeability-surface area product (**H**) only has a slight rim of high K2 in the periphery of the lesion. This is because so much contrast agent is present that the T2 effects outweigh the T1 effects during the perfusion scan and therefore the degree of change there is outside the scope of the correction algorithm. See also Movie Clip ⊙ **31** for documentation of the change in signal in the meningioma; compare with the infarct in the basal ganglia. Pathological analysis of the extra-axial lesion demonstrated a malignant meningioma.

Direction of biopsy/intervention

Low grade lesions have a typical appearance on conventional MRI. However, on occasion lesions which appear low grade on conventional pre- and post-contrast MR studies can have focal areas of malignant dedifferentiation; perfusion MRI may be able to highlight such areas. Figs. **47** and **48** demonstrate how rCBV maps can be used to aid in determining where to biopsy or treat these lesions. In each of these cases, the conventional MRI demonstrated a relatively homogeneous appearance, even after the administration of intravenous contrast agent. However, the rCBV and PET studies demonstrate focal areas of increased signal corresponding to higher grade tumor. The rCBV maps can be used not only to direct the surgical biopsy but can also occasionally directly aid the pathologist. Fig. **49** demonstrates a case in which the original pathology reading was based on only some of the surgical samples (taken outside the area of high rCBV) and was reported as low grade astrocytoma. After review of the rCBV map, which clearly showed regions of intense microvascular proliferation suggesting greater malignancy, additional tissue specimens were located from surgical samples localized to the rCBV "hot" areas. These samples subsequently documented the lesion as high-grade.

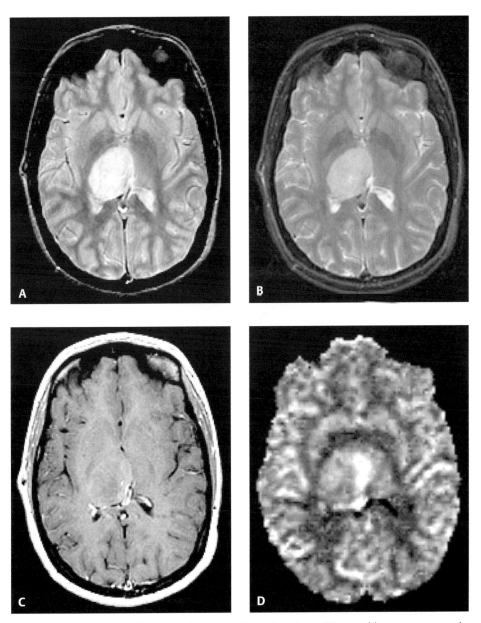

Fig. **47**   Heterogeneity of glioma seen best on perfusion imaging. A 26-year-old woman presented with headache and right-sided weakness.

Proton density-weighted (**A**), T2-weighted (**B**), and T1-post-contrast imaging (**C**) demonstrate minimal enhancement and overall homogeneous signal.

The rCBV (**D**) demonstrates focal high rCBV in the medial aspect of the lesion. Biopsy of this area demonstrated grade III/IV astrocytoma (from [138], courtesy of B. Rosen/H. Aronen).

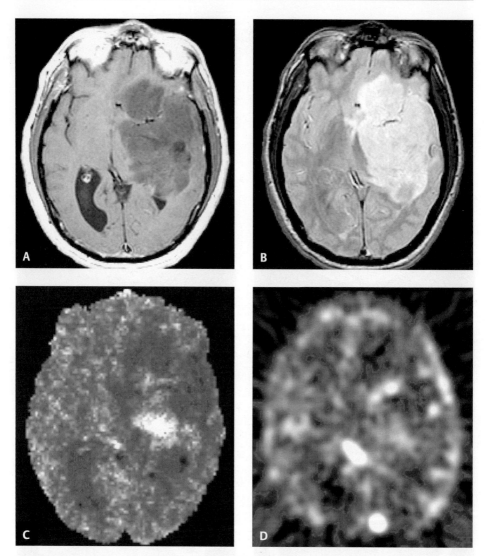

Fig. 48 Heterogeneity of glioma seen best on rCBV maps in a 51-year-old male.

(A) A post-contrast T1-weighted image shows marked mass effect but little enhancement.
(B) The T2-weighted image shows a fairly homogeneous mass.
(C) The rCBV map demonstrates a focus of high rCBV.

(D) CBV measurement with PET [11]CO confirms the location of this high CBV region, suggesting a more malignant focus of dedifferentiation. Subsequent biopsy showed that this focus was indeed malignant (from Sorensen AG, Rosen B 1996 [138]).

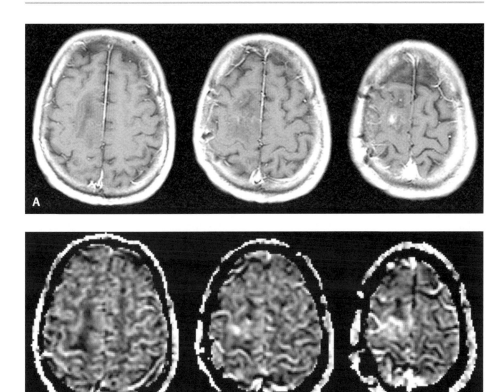

Fig. **49**   A 57-year-old man presented 7 years after resection of an oligodendroglioma.

(**A**) Post-contrast T1-weighted images (top row) demonstrate slight enhancement in the area of prior surgery.

(**B**) Maps of rCBV (bottom row) demonstrate an area of high rCBV approximately 2 cm anterior to the central sulcus. Biopsies from in front and behind the area of highest rCBV demonstrated low grade tumor, and a biopsy in the lesion in the area of highest rCBV demonstrated grade 3/4 astrocytoma (from Sorensen AG, Rosen B 1996 [138]).

Treatment follow-up

A hallmark of gliomas is that they are extremely infiltrative. The margins are difficult to define even at pathology and autopsy [106]. As a result, surgical procedures are rarely curative, but rather cytoreductive, and are combined with radiation and chemotherapy. As a result, follow-up studies are typically obtained at three- and six-month intervals to rule out "recurrence." Of course, since some tumor has almost invariably been left behind, the question is not about microscopic levels of slow-growing tumor, but rather whether or not rapidly growing, highly malignant foci are present. The questions for evaluation via follow-up imaging also include the effectiveness of the radiotherapy and/or the detection of invasion or malignant degeneration in previously low-grade lesions. In particular, radiation often has a delayed effect, causing mass lesions with enhancement six to twelve months or more after completion of therapy. While conventional MRI depends on blood-brain barrier destruction and on changes in serial imaging studies, such markers are often nonspecific, and it is frequently impossible to distinguish radionecrosis from recurrence on conventional MRI alone. While a number of studies have suggested other approaches such as PET or SPECT, these have been limited and occasionally contradictory [71]. The distinction between radiation necrosis and bulk tumor recurrence is particularly difficult with conventional MRI or CT, since both tumor and radiation necrosis can show blood-brain barrier breakdown, mass effect, and edema. Perfusion MRI, specifically rCBV mapping may be able to furnish this same distinction, provided that the rCBV maps are made with care. Such care includes the need for pre-dosing with Gd before performing the injection, since a leaky BBB is almost always present.

Fig. **50** demonstrates a case of short-term follow-up studies after radiotherapy. Figs. **51**, **52**, and **53** demonstrate rCBV mapping in biopsy-proven recurrence. Fig. **54** demonstrates biopsy-proven radiation necrosis. Our own experience has demonstrated some success with rCBV. For example, in 15 cases where there was a clinical and radiological question of radiation necrosis versus tumor recurrence which went to biopsy after rCBV mapping, that rCBV mapping was able to correctly predict the absence or presence of tumor in 14 of 15 cases [107]. Note that in the radiated areas of the brain, rCBV is typically lower than normal. This is probably due to the effect of radiation on the capillary bed. Some studies have identified reductions in rCBV after radiation [108] as well as after normal aging [109] and chemotherapy [110].

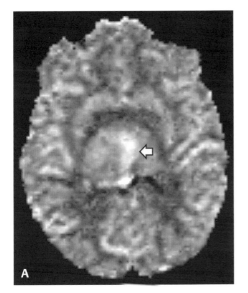

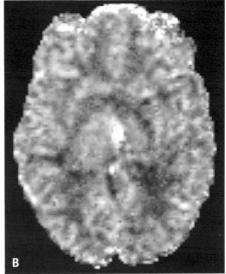

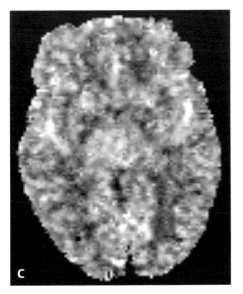

Fig. **50**   Relative CBV mapping of response to therapy. Same patient as in Fig. **47**.

Mapping of rCBV pre-radiation (**A**), 6 weeks after radiation (**B**), and 5 months post-radiation (**C**) demonstrate gradual decrease in rCBV, consistent with radiation effect on the microvasculature.

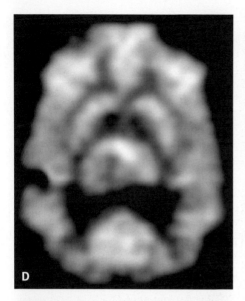

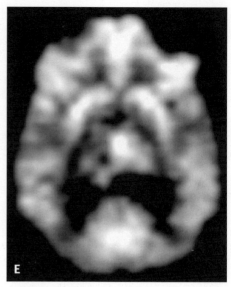

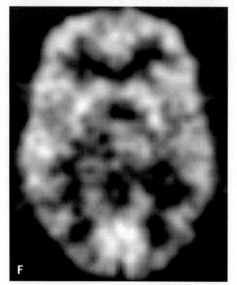

50   There was also decrease in PET [18] FDG uptake, shown again pre-radiation (**D**), 6 weeks after radiation (**E**), and 5 months out (**F**) (from Sorensen AG, Rosen B 1996 [138]).

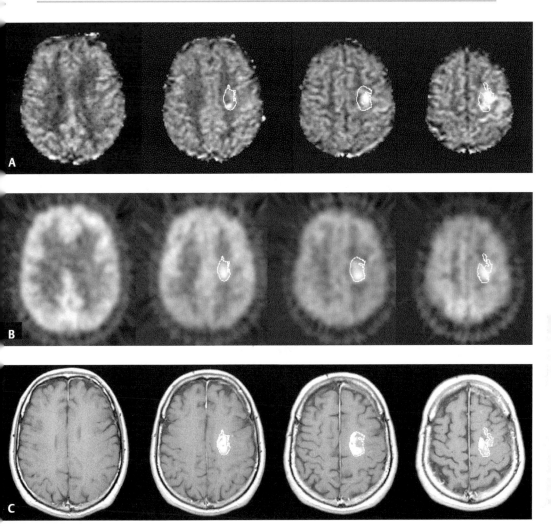

Fig. **51**   High grade tumor.

A 47-year-old man demonstrates a bright focus of rCBV (**A**), which is confirmed as high uptake on the PET ^{18}FDG study (**B**).

Post-contrast T1-weighted imaging (**C**) demonstrated a slightly larger area of enhancement than the area of high CBV or high PET ^{18}FDG uptake. Biopsy showed anaplastic mixed glioma/oligodendroglioma, grade III/IV (from Sorensen AG, Rosen B 1996 [138]).

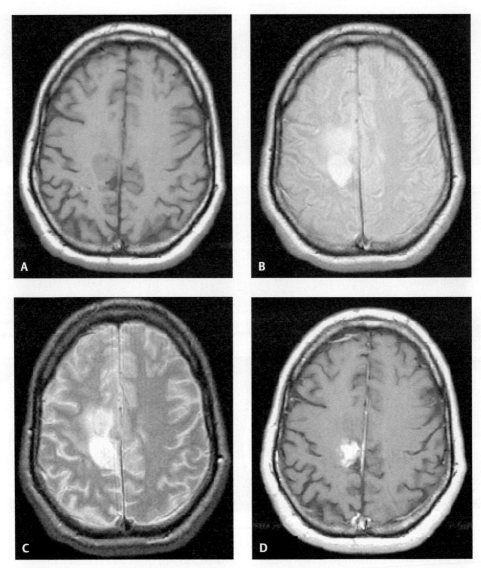

Fig. 52   Anaplastic astrocytoma. A 47-year-old male with a known low-grade oligodendroglioma presents with new enhancement on post-contrast T1-weighted images.

Pre-contrast T1-weighted imaging (**A**), proton-density weighted imaging (**B**), T2 (**C**) and

T1-post Gd imaging (**D**) demonstrate an area of enhancement with surrounding edema.

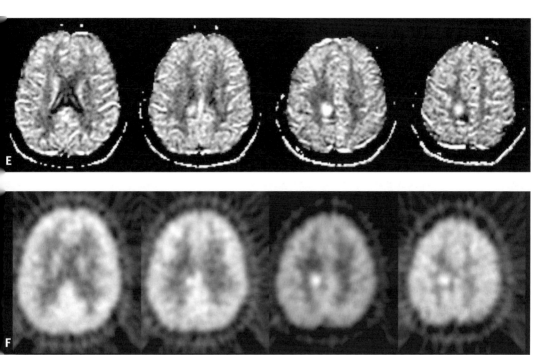

52 rCBV maps (**E**) and PET ¹⁸FDG (**F**) both show high signal in the region, consistent with either a high capillary count (rCBV) or high metabolism (PET), both suggestive of a high-grade lesion (from Sorensen AG, Rosen B 1996 [138]).

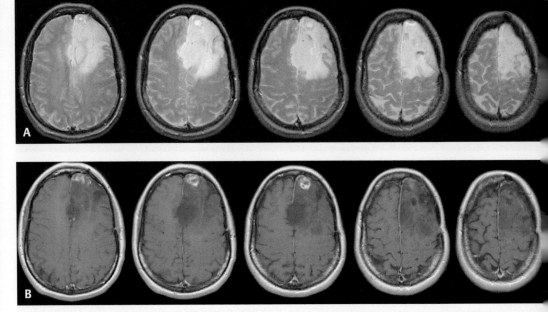

Fig. 53 Recurrence post-radiation in a 34-year-old woman 6 years after excision and radiation of a low-grade astrocytoma.

(A) T2-weighted images demonstrate a diffuse T2 abnormality consistent with radiation effect or tumor.

(B) Post-Gd T1-weighted images show a focus of enhancement in a ring-like fashion. This is still not specific for radiation or recurrence.

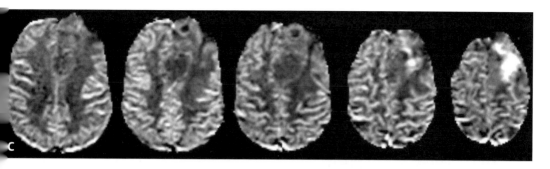

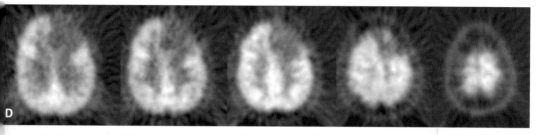

53   (**C**) Maps of rCBV demonstrate only mildly increased rCBV in the enhancing area, but markedly increased rCBV more cranially. Biopsy showed malignant mixed glioma.

(**D**) PET [18]FDG showed increased glucose uptake near the vertex, though not quite as clearly as the rCBV maps (from Sorensen AG, Rosen B 1996 [138]).

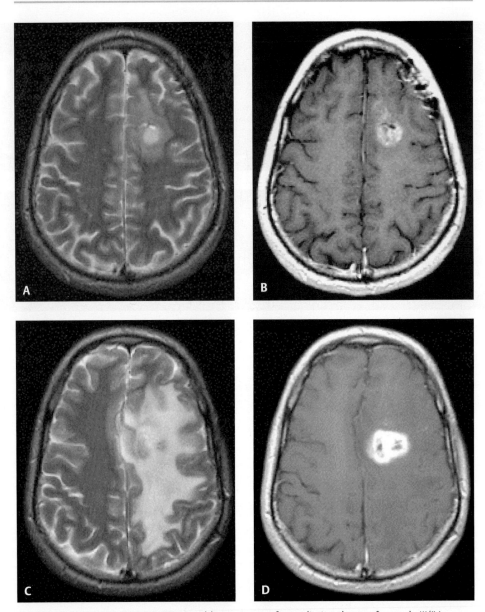

Fig. **54** Radiation necrosis in a 42-year-old man 1 year after radiation therapy for grade III/IV astrocytoma.

T2 (**A**) and T1-post-contrast (**B**) images six months after surgery show a small lesion. The same sequences performed six months later

(**C** and **D**) demonstrate increased T2 signal abnormality, increased enhancement, and greater mass effect.

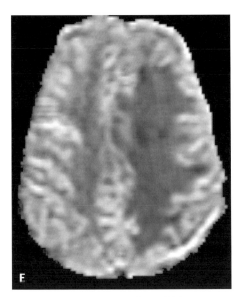 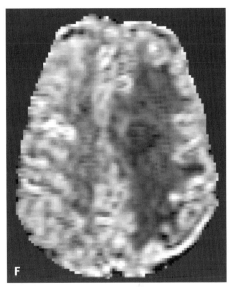

54   Maps of rCBV using either Gd (**E**) or Dy-DTPA-BMA (**F**) demonstrate no areas of rCBV greater than the contralateral (and pre- sumably normal) white matter. Biopsy showed radiation effect without tumor (from Sorensen AG, Rosen B 1996 [138]).

In summary, perfusion mapping of tumors can add to the diagnosis and management of patients with primary CNS malignancies. Because these studies can be performed as additions to conventional MR evaluations with little added time, they may serve as a cost effective alternative to radionuclide-based functional imaging studies. Although additional data on the ultimate clinical utility of these techniques are needed, the primary advantages of low incremental costs combined with high anatomic resolution and the ability to easily register functional images with anatomic images from a single modality make it likely that these methods will find increasing use.

Dementia

Dementia is one of the most common diseases and yet one quite difficult to diagnose radiographically. The most common subtype, senile dementia of the Alzheimer type (SDAT) remains particularly challenging. PET studies have shown some success in this setting [111], with characteristic decreases in [18] FDG uptake in moderate to severe cases of SDAT. Recent PET work has also shown decreases in rCBV, rCBF, and increases in the oxygen extraction fraction [112]. Perfusion imaging with fMRI has been applied to this problem as well, with early studies indicating similar results to those of PET [113] and SPECT [114,115,]. These early studies indicate that fMRI rCBV mapping may have a sensitivity and specificity similar to that of nuclear medicine approaches for the diagnosis of SDAT. A typical case is illustrated in Fig. 55.

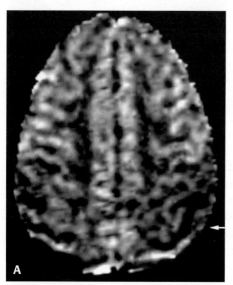 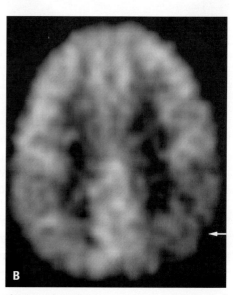

Fig. 55   Dementia. This patient with Alzheimer's disease demonstrates decreased rCBV in the parietal lobe (arrow, **A**) and also decreased uptake of [8] FDG on a PET study.

This is a relatively common pattern of decreased blood volume and metabolism in AD (from Sorensen AG, Rosen B 1996 [138]. Courtesy of R. G. Gonzalez).

Vascular causes of dementia have been evaluated with perfusion MRI. These studies have shown that rCBV tends to be below normal, particularly in white matter[116], and in some cases even lower than in SDAT[117]. Other approaches to imaging diagnosis of Alzheimer's include observing fMRI activation mapping during neuropsychiatric testing of memory formation and retrieval[118], which may be apparent earlier than the structural changes associated with changes in lobar blood volume. As in many other areas of clinical application, these studies are still in progress.

Vasospasm

Subarachnoid hemorrhage is followed by vasospasm in up to 70% of patients, usually occurring within 10 days after aneurysm rupture. These patients can be difficult to monitor because they are often neurologically impaired at baseline, either due to the consequences of the ruptured aneurysm or occasionally because of corrective surgery. Perfusion MRI has been shown to be sensitive to the abnormalities present in vasospasm. Fig. **56** shows an example of this, highlighting how marked the abnormalities can be. Interestingly, here again there are almost certainly technical artifacts present because of inaccurate local arterial input functions. The diffuse abnormality in the arteries and arterioles is bound to alter the local AIF. Quantitative CBF is difficult in such cases, even with PET because the assumption that the radial artery AIF is equal to the MCA AIF is equal to the local voxel's AIF breaks down. Nevertheless, the ability to document disturbances even nonspecifically may still help guide clinical treatment. We know that timing maps such as arrival time, from the purist's view, may not be physiologically meaningful in the same way true MTT has a defined physiological meaning, even so, such maps can still identify areas of abnormal hemodynamics and can play a (carefully restricted) role in clinical management. Similarly, PWI-based (or even PET-based) MTT or rCBF maps may not actually be accurate due to the local pathology, but still might be useful in patient management decisions.

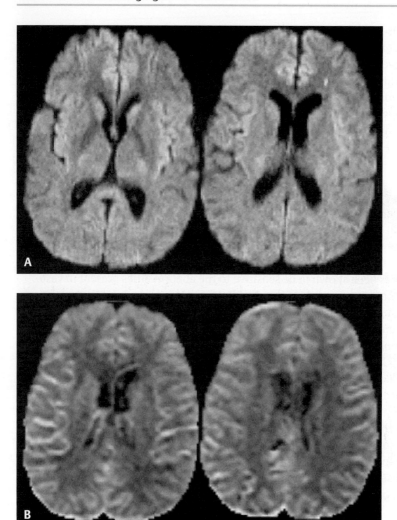

Fig. 56   Vasospasm. A 33-year-old male with symptomatic vasospasm after subarachnoid hemorrhage.

Diffusion-weighted images (**A**) demonstrate no clear abnormality, while CBV (**B**), CBF (**C**), and MTT (**D**) images demonstrate extensive abnormal signal in the left hemisphere.

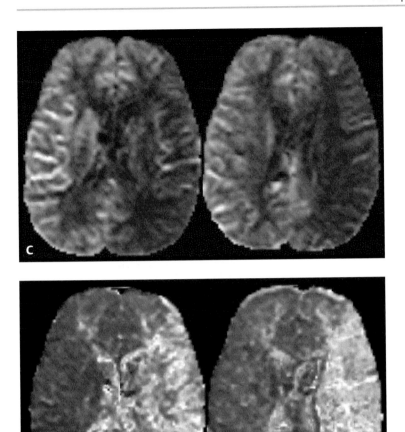

56 The patient was subsequently treated with hypervolemia and hypertension with good outcome. Some of the perfusion abnormality could be due to delay and dispersion as discussed above. See also Movie Clip ⊙ **32**.

Head trauma

Perfusion imaging may have a major role to play in trauma, since many hypothesize that the damage from head trauma comes from alterations in blood flow rather than from direct energy deposition. As with ischemic stroke, imaging early after the onset of symptoms may be key to detecting these abnormalities. To date, imaging has been limited to the subacute period, and therefore imaging findings have not been widely used to direct therapy. Nevertheless, there are perfusion defects in human trauma, and perfusion MRI appears to have the sensitivity needed to find them. Fig. **57** demonstrates an example of such a lesion. Trauma is a major cause of morbidity, with accidents being the leading cause of death in the 15- to 44-year age range in the United States in 1996 [119]. This is an excellent example of a disease where perfusion imaging may be able to help us understand an illness that is currently largely without effective treatments.

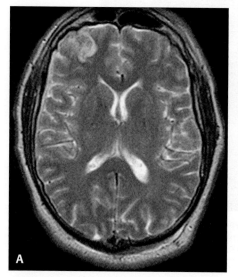
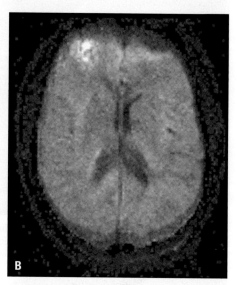

Fig. **57**   Trauma in a 29-year-old male. T2-weighted images (**A**) and DWI (**B**) demonstrate a focus of bright signal in the right frontal lobe, consistent with tissue damage due to direct energy deposition.

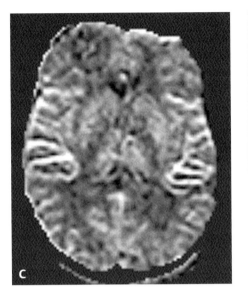

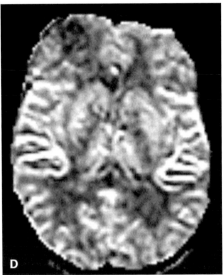

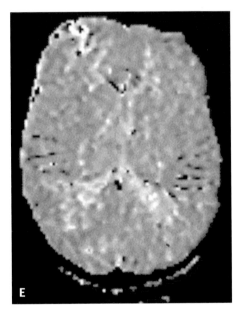

57 Perfusion images show a larger area of abnormality, as seen on CBV (**C**), CBF (**D**), and MTT (**E**). See also Movie Clip ⊙ **33**.

Migraine

Perfusion abnormalities have been reported in a variety of phases of migraine. Because the migraine aura precedes the actual headache, substantial work has been focused on the study of this phase of the migraine. Cutrer et al. have reported perfusion defects with perfusion MRI that are similar to case reports using other modalities [120]. An example of this is shown in Fig. **58**. It appears that these abnormalities spread from an initial area. While perfusion defects are likely not the primary pathophysiological event in migraine, the ability of perfusion MRI to document such abnormalities highlights some of its benefits.

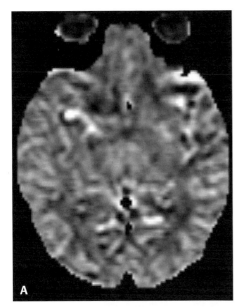

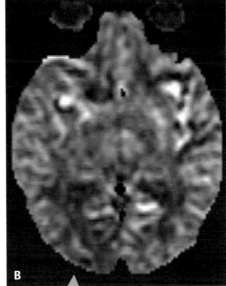

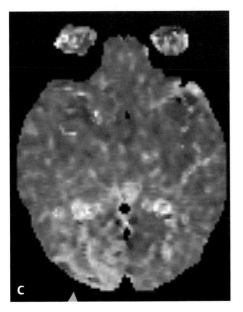

Fig. **58** Migraine. Perfusion defects in a 36-year-old male with left hemianopia.

CBV (**A**), CBF (**B**), and MTT (**C**) all demonstrate abnormal perfusion in the right occipital lobe, in the retinotopically appropriate location. See also Movie Clip ⊙ **34**.

Epilepsy

Because fMRI does not yet visualize neuronal firing, but rather the hemodynamic changes associated with neural activity, seizures are best identified ictally [121,122]. An ictal MR image is shown in Fig. 59. However, this is impractical, and most imaging is done interictally. Often an anatomic abnormality can be found.

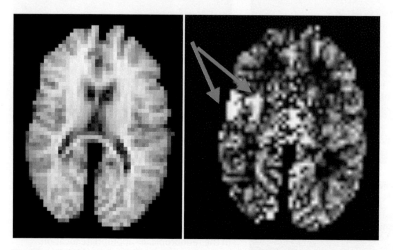

Fig. **59**   High blood flow in a patient with epilepsy studied with a non-contrast technique (FAIR). The image on the left is the T1-weighted baseline image, created with an echo-planar technique. On the right is the image of CBF, indicating an area of high flow in the focus of presumed seizure activity (figure courtesy K. Kwong).

The most common cause of partial complex seizures is mesial temporal sclerosis [123]. Early studies comparing PET and rCBV mapping suggest that rCBV can demonstrate lateralizing findings, showing decreased rCBV in hippocampal atrophy and increased rCBV during ictus [124].

Other lesions

Perfusion MRI has been used to study a variety of other conditions. Reports of rCBV elevation in patients with HIV [125], rCBV changes after psychotropic medications [126], hypercapnia [127], or cocaine [128,129] have been published. Perfusion MRI has also been used to study cerebral hemodynamics in patients with intraparenchymal hemorrhage [130], sickle cell anemia [131], schizophrenia [132], and in patients undergoing evaluation of cerebrovascular reserve [133–135]. It may be that other subtle pharmacological interventions will be measurable with perfusion MRI studies [136].

Conclusion

Perfusion MRI can potentially bring a series of new patient populations and disease entities to the radiologist. Understanding the technical issues of perfusion as well as the underlying cerebral physiology and pathophysiology is necessary to bring the full benefit of these techniques to patient care. Currently, perfusion imaging appears to provide benefit to patients in the evaluation of neoplasm and stroke; other areas are under active investigation.

References

Selected reading

Perfusion methodology

Calamante F, Thomas DL, Pell GS, Wiersma J, Turner R. Measuring cerebral blood flow using magnetic resonance imaging techniques. J Cereb Blood Flow Metab 1999; 19:701–735.

Emerson JF, Chen PC, Shankle WR, Haier RJ, Nalcioglu O. Data analysis for dynamic contrast-enhanced MRI-based cerebral perfusion measurements: correcting for changing cortical CSF volumes. Magma 1995; 3(1): 41–48.

Heiland S, Benner T, Debus J, Rempp K, Reith W, Sartor K. Simultaneous assessment of cerebral hemodynamics and contrast agent uptake in lesions with disrupted blood-brain-barrier. Magn Reson Imaging 1999; 17(1): 21–27.

Heiland S, Kreibich W, Reith W, Benner T, Dorfler A, Forsting M, Sartor K. Comparison of echo-planar sequences for perfusion-weighted MRI: which is best? Neuro-radiology 1998; 40(4): 216–221.

Jezzard P. Advances in perfusion MR imaging. Radiology 1998; 208:296–299.

Kauczor H, Surkau R, Roberts T. MRI using hyperpolarized noble gases. Eur Radiol 1998; 8(5): 820–827.

Lev MH, Kulke SF, Sorensen AG, Boxerman JL, Brady TJ, Rosen BR, Buchbinder BR, Weisskoff RM. Contrast-to-noise ratio in functional MRI of relative cerebral blood volume with sprodiamide injection. J Magn Reson Imaging 1997; 7:523–527.

Reimer P, Schuierer G, Balzer T. Peters PE. Application of a superparamagnetic iron oxide (Resovist) for MR imaging of human cerebral blood volume. Magn Reson Med 1995; 34(5): 694–697.

Rempp KA, Brix G, Wenz FRBC, Gückel F, Lorenz WJ. Quantification of regional cerebral blood flow and volume with dynamic susceptibility contrast-enhanced MR imaging. Radiology 1994; 193:637–641.

Rostrup E, Larsson HB, Toft PB, Garde K, Ring PB, Henriksen O. Susceptibility contrast imaging of CO_2-induced changes in the blood volume of the human brain. Acta Radiol 1996; 37(5): 813–822.

Runge VM, Kirsch JE, Wells JW, Woolfolk CE. Assessment of cerebral perfusion by first-pass, dynamic, contrast-enhanced, steady-state free-precession MR imaging: an animal study. Am J Roentgenol 1993; 160(3): 593–600.

Speck O, Chang L, Itti L, Itti E, Ernst T. Comparison of static and dynamic MRI techniques for the measurement of regional cerebral blood volume. Magn Reson Med 1999; 41(6): 1264–1268.

Unger EC, Ugurbil K, Latchaw RE. Contrast agents for cerebral perfusion MR imaging. J Magn Reson Imaging 1994; 4(3): 235 – 242.

Clinical applications: ischemia

Adams WM, Laitt RD, Li KL, Jackson A, Sherrington CR, Talbot P. Demonstration of cerebral perfusion abnormalities in moyamoya disease using susceptibility perfusion- and diffusion-weighted MRI. Neuroradiology 1999; 41(2): 86 – 92.

Ay H, Buonanno FS, Rordorf G, Schaefer PW, Schwamm LH, Wu O, Gonzalez RG, Yamada K, Sorensen GA, et al. Normal diffusion-weighted MRI during stroke-like deficits. Neurology 1999; 52(9): 1784 – 1792.

Baird AE, Benfield A, Schlaug G, Siewert B, Lovblad KO, Edelman RR, Warach S. Enlargement of human cerebral ischemic lesion volumes measured by diffusion-weighted magnetic resonance imaging. Ann Neurol 1997; 41(5): 581 – 589.

Berthezene Y, Nighoghossian N, Damien J, Derex L, Trouillas P, Froment JC. Effects of thalamic hemorrhage on cortical hemodynamic parameters assessed by perfusion MR imaging: preliminary report. J Neurol Sci 1998; 157(1): 67 – 72.

Berthezene Y, Nighoghossian N, Meyer R, Damien J, Cinotti L, Adeleine P, Trouillas P, Froment JC. Can cerebrovascular reactivity be assessed by dynamic susceptibility contrast-enhanced MRI? Neuroradiology 1998; 40(1): 1 – 5.

Bitzer M, Klose U, Nagele T, Friese S, Kuntz R, Fetter M, Opitz H, Voigt K. (1999). Echo planar perfusion imaging with high spatial and temporal resolution: methodology and clinical aspects. Eur Radiol 1999; 9(2): 221 – 229.

Fisher M, Albers GW. Applications of diffusion-perfusion magnetic resonance imaging in acute ischemic stroke]. Neurology 1999; 52(9): 1750 – 1756.

Karonen JO, Vanninen RL, Liu Y, Østergaard L, Kuikka JT, Nuutinen J, Vanninen EJ, Partanen PL, Vainio PA, et al. Combined diffusion and perfusion MRI with correlation to single-photon emission CT in acute ischemic stroke: ischemic penumbra predicts infarct growth. Stroke 1999; 30(8): 1583 – 1590.

Keller E, Flacke S, Urbach H, Schild HH. Diffusion- and perfusion-weighted magnetic resonance imaging in deep cerebral venous thrombosis. Stroke 1999; 30(5): 1144 – 1146.

Kim JH, Shin T, Park JH, Chung SH, Choi NC, Lim BH. Various patterns of perfusion-weighted MR imaging and MR angiographic findings in hyperacute ischemic stroke. Am J Neuroradiol 1999; 20(4): 613 – 620.

Kluytmans M, van der Grond J, Folkers PJ, Mali MP, Viergever MA. Differentiation of gray matter and white matter perfusion in patients with unilateral internal carotid artery occlusion. J Magn Reson Imaging 1998; 8(4): 767 – 774.

Maeda M, Maley JE, Crosby DL, Quets JP, Zhu MW, Lee GJ, Lawler GJ, Ueda T, Bendixen BH, et al. Application of contrast agents in the evaluation of stroke: conventional MR and echo-planar MR imaging. J Magn Reson Imaging 1997; 7(1): 23 – 28.

Maeda M, Yuh WT, Ueda T, Maley JE, Crosby DL, Zhu MW, Magnotta VA. Severe occlusive carotid artery disease: hemodynamic assessment by MR perfusion imaging in symptomatic patients. Am J Neuroradiol 1999; 20(1): 43 – 51.

Nighoghossian N, Berthezene Y, Adeleine P, Wiart M, Damien J, Derex L, Itti R, Froment JC, Trouillas P. Effects of subcortical cerebrovascular lesions on cortical hemodynamic parameters assessed by perfusion magnetic resonance imaging. Cerebrovasc Dis 1999; 9(3): 136 – 141.

Nighoghossian N, Berthezene Y, Meyer R, Cinotti L, Adeleine P, Philippon B, Froment JC, Trouillas P. Assessment of cerebrovascular reactivity by dynamic susceptibility contrast-enhanced MR imaging. J Neurol Sci 1997; 149(2): 171 – 176.

Oppenheimer SM, Bryan RN, Conturo TE, Soher BJ, Preziosi TJ, Barker PB. Proton magnetic resonance spectroscopy and gadolinium-DTPA perfusion imaging of asymptomatic MRI white matter lesions. Magn Reson Med 1995; 33(1): 61 – 68.

Reith W, Heiland S, Erb G, Benner T, Forsting M, Sartor K. Dynamic contrast-enhanced T2*-weighted MRI in patients with cerebrovascular disease. Neuroradiology 1997; 39(4): 250 – 257.

Rordorf G, Koroshetz WJ, Copen WA, Cramer SC, Schaefer PW, Budzik Jr, RF, Schwamm LH, Buonanno F, Sorensen AG, et al. Regional ischemia and ischemic injury in patients with acute middle cerebral artery stroke as defined by early diffusion-weighted and perfusion-weighted MRI. Stroke 1998; 29(5): 939 – 943.

Rordorf G, Koroshetz WJ, Copen WA, Gonzalez G, Yamada K, Schaefer PW, Schwamm LH, Ogilvy CS, Sorensen AG. Diffusion- and perfusion-weighted imaging in vasospasm after subarachnoid hemorrhage. Stroke 1999; 30(3): 599 – 605.

Rowe J, Blamire AM, Domingo Z, Moody V, Molyneux A, Byrne J, Cadoux-Hudson T, Radda G. Discrepancies between cerebral perfusion and metabolism after subarachnoid haemorrhage: a magnetic resonance approach. J Neurol Neurosurg Psychiatry 1998; 64(1): 98 – 103.

Sorensen AG, Wray SH, Weisskoff RM, Boxerman JL, Davis TL, Caramia F, Kwong KK, Stern CE, Baker JR, et al. Functional MR of brain activity and perfusion in patients with chronic cortical stroke. Am J Neuroradiol 1995; 16(9): 1753 – 1762.

Tsuchida C, Yamada H, Maeda M, Sadato N, Matsuda T, Kawamura Y, Hayashi N, Yamamoto K, Yonekura Y, et al. Evaluation of peri-infarcted hypoperfusion with T2*-weighted dynamic MRI. J Magn Reson Imaging 1997; 7(3): 518 – 522.

Tsuchiya K, Inaoka S, Mizutani Y, Hachiya J. Echo-planar perfusion MR of moyamoya disease. Am J Neuroradiol 1998; 19(2): 211 – 216.

Warach S, Dashe JF, Edelman RR. Clinical outcome in ischemic stroke predicted by early diffusion-weighted and perfusion magnetic resonance imaging: a preliminary analysis. J Cereb Blood Flow Metab 1996; 16(1): 53 – 59.

Wu RH, Bruening R, Berchtenbreiter C, Weber J, Steiger HJ, Peller M, Penzkofer H, Reiser M. MRI assessment of cerebral blood volume in patients with brain infarcts. Neuroradiology 1998; 40(8): 496 – 502.

Clinical applications: tumors

Domingo Z, Rowe G, Blamire AM, Cadoux-Hudson TA. Role of ischaemia in the genesis of oedema surrounding meningiomas assessed using magnetic resonance imaging and spectroscopy. Br J Neurosurg 1998; 12(5): 414–418.

Ernst TM, Chang L, Witt MD, Aronow HA, Cornford ME, Walot I, Goldberg MA. Cerebral toxoplasmosis and lymphoma in AIDS: perfusion MR imaging experience in 13 patients. Radiology 1998; 208(3): 663–669.

Knopp EA, Cha S, Johnson G, Mazumdar A, Golfinos JG, Zagzag D, Miller DC, Kelly PJ, Kricheff II. Glial neoplasms: dynamic contrast-enhanced T2*-weighted MR imaging. Radiology 1999; 211(3): 791–798.

Siegal T, Rubinstein R, Tzuk-Shina T. Gomori JM. Utility of relative cerebral blood volume mapping derived from perfusion magnetic resonance imaging in the routine follow up of brain tumors. J Neurosurg 1997; 86(1): 22–27.

Sugahara T, Korogi Y, Kochi M, Ikushima I, Hirai T, Okuda T, Shigematsu Y, Liang L, Ge Y, et al. Correlation of MR imaging-determined cerebral blood volume maps with histologic and angiographic determination of vascularity of gliomas. Am J Roentgenol 1998; 171(6): 1479–1486.

Sugahara T, Korogi Y, Shigematsu Y, Hirai T, Ikushima I, Liang L, Ushio Y, Takahashi M. Perfusion-sensitive MRI of cerebral lymphomas: a preliminary report. J Comput Assist Tomogr 1999; 23(2): 232–237.

Wenz F, Rempp K, Hess T, Debus J, Brix G, Engenhart R, Knopp M V, van Kaick G, Wannenmacher M. Effect of radiation on blood volume in low-grade astrocytomas and normal brain tissue: quantification with dynamic susceptibility contrast MR imaging. Am J Roentgenol 1996; 166: 187–193.

Clinical applications: other areas

Ernst T, Chang L, Itti L, Speck O. Correlation of regional cerebral blood flow from perfusion MRI and SPECT in normal subjects. Magn Reson Imaging 1999; 17(3): 349–354.

Hagen T, Bartylla K, Piepgras U. Correlation of regional cerebral blood flow measured by stable xenon CT and perfusion MRI. J Comput Assist Tomogr 1999; 23(2): 257–264.

Levin JM, Ross MH, Harris G, Renshaw PF. Applications of dynamic susceptibility contrast magnetic resonance imaging in neuropsychiatry. Neuroimage 1996; 4: 147–162.

Renshaw PF, Levin JM, Kaufman MJ, Ross MH, Lewis RF, Harris GJ. Dynamic susceptibility contrast magnetic resonance imaging in neuropsychiatry: present utility and future promise. Eur Radiol 1997; 7(Suppl 5): 216–221.

Sheth TN, Ichise M, Kucharczyk W. Brain perfusion imaging in asymptomatic patients receiving cyclosporin. Am J Neuroradiol 1999; 20(5): 853–856.

Sorensen AG, Tievsky AL, Østergaard L, Weisskoff RM, Rosen BR. Contrast agents in functional MR imaging. J Magn Reson Imaging 1997; 7(1): 47–55.

Stoll M, Hagen T, Bartylla K, Weber M, Jost V, Treib J. Changes of cerebral perfusion after osmotherapy in acute cerebral edema assessed with perfusion weighted MRI. Neurol Res 1998; 20(6): 474–478.

Yuh WT, Ueda T, Maley JE. Perfusion and diffusion imaging: a potential tool for improved diagnosis of CNS vasculitis. Am J Neuroradiol 1999; 20(1): 87–89.

Wenz F, Rempp K, Brix G, Knopp MV, Guckel F, Hess T, van Kaick G. Age dependency of the regional cerebral blood volume (rCBV) measured with dynamic susceptibility contrast MR imaging (DSC). Magnetic Resonance Imaging 1996; 14: 157–162.

Non-contrast perfusion methodology

Crelier GR, Hoge RD, Munger P, Pike GB. Perfusion-based functional magnetic resonance imaging with single-shot RARE and GRASE acquisitions. Magn Reson Med 1999; 41(1): 132–136.

Detre JA, Alsop DC. Perfusion magnetic resonance imaging with continuous arterial spin labeling: methods and clinical applications in the central nervous system. Eur J Radiol 1999; 30 (2): 115–124.

Detre JA, Leigh JS, Williams DS, Koretsky AP. (1992). Perfusion imaging. Magn Reson Med 1992; 23(1): 37–45.

Tanabe JL, Yongbi M, Branch C, Hrabe J, Johnson G, Helpern JA. MR perfusion imaging in human brain using the UNFAIR technique. Un-inverted flow-sensitive alternating inversion recovery. J Magn Reson Imaging 1999; 9(6): 761–767.

Wong EC, Buxton RB, Frank LR. Quantitative perfusion imaging using arterial spin labeling. Neuroimaging Clin N Am 1999; 9(2): 333–342.

Yang Y, Frank JA, Hou L, Ye FQ, McLaughlin AC, Duyn JH. Multislice imaging of quantitative cerebral perfusion with pulsed arterial spin labeling. Magn Reson Med 1998; 39 (5): 825–832.

Ye FQ, Pekar JJ, Jezzard P, Duyn J, Frank JA, McLaughlin AC. Perfusion imaging of the human brain at 1.5 T using a single-shot EPI spin tagging approach. Magn Reson Med 1996; 36(2): 217–224.

Perfusion MRI in animal studies

Calamante F, Lythgoe MF, Pell GS, Thomas DL, King MD, Busza AL, Sotak CH, Williams SR, Ordidge RJ, et al. Early changes in water diffusion, perfusion, T1, and T2 during focal cerebral ischemia in the rat studied at 8.5 T. Magn Reson Med 1999; 41(3): 479–485.

D'Arceuil HE, de Crespigny AJ, Rother J, Seri S, Moseley ME, Stevenson DK, Rhine W. Diffusion and perfusion magnetic resonance imaging of the evolution of hypoxic ischemic encephalopathy in the neonatal rabbit. J Magn Reson Imaging 1998; 8(4): 820–828.

Dijkhuizen RM, Berkelbach van der Sprenkel JW, Tulleken WA, Nicolay K. Regional assessment of tissue oxygenation and the temporal evolution of hemodynamic parameters and water diffusion during acute focal ischemia in rat brain. Brain Res 1997; 750(1,2): 161–170.

Doerfler A, Forsting M, Reith W, Heiland S, Weber J, Hacke W, Sartor K. Bolus injection of MR contrast agents: hemodynamic effects evaluated by intracerebral laser Doppler flowmetry in rats. Am J Neuroradiol 1997; 18(3): 427–434.

Forbes ML, Hendrich KS, Kochanek PM, Williams DS, Schiding JK, Wisniewski SR, Kelsey SF, DeKosky ST, Graham SH, et al. Assessment of cerebral blood flow and CO_2 reactivity after controlled cortical impact by perfusion magnetic resonance imaging using arterial spin-labeling in rats [published erratum appears in J Cereb Blood Flow Metab 1997; 17(11): 1263]. J Cereb Blood Flow Metab 1997; 17(8): 865–874.

Haraldseth O, Jones RA, Muller TB, Fahlvik AK; Oksendal AN. Comparison of dysprosium DTPA BMA and superparamagnetic iron oxide particles as susceptibility contrast agents for perfusion imaging of regional cerebral ischemia in the rat. J Magn Reson Imaging 1996; 6(5): 714–717.

Hossmann KA, Hoehn-Berlage M. Diffusion and perfusion MR imaging of cerebral ischemia. Cerebrovasc Brain Metab Rev 1995; 7(3): 187–217.

Knight RA, Barker PB, Fagan SC, Li Y, Jacobs MA, Welch KM. Prediction of impending hemorrhagic transformation in ischemic stroke using magnetic resonance imaging in rats. Stroke 1998; 29(1): 144–151.

Rother J, de Crespigny AJ, D'Arceuil H, Iwai K, Moseley ME. Recovery of apparent diffusion coefficient after ischemia-induced spreading depression relates to cerebral perfusion gradient. Stroke 1996; 27(5): 980–986; discussion 986–987.

Simonesen CZ, Østergaard L, Vestergaard-Poulsen P, Rohl L, Bjornerud A, Gyldensted C. CBF and CBV measurements by USPIO bolus tracking: reproducibility and comparison with Gd-based values. J Magn Reson Imaging 1999; 9(2): 342–347.

Zaharchuk G, Bogdanov Jr, AA, Marota JJ, Shimizu-Sasamata M, Weisskoff RM, Kwong KK, Jenkins BG, Weissleder R, Rosen BR. Continuous assessment of perfusion by tagging including volume and water extraction (CAPTIVE): a steady-state contrast agent technique for measuring blood flow, relative blood volume fraction, and the water extraction fraction. Magn Reson Med 1998; 40(5): 666–678.

Cited papers

[1]   Rosen BR, Belliveau JW, Aronen HJ, Kennedy D, Buchbinder BR, Fischman A, Gruber M, Glas J, Weisskoff RM, Cohen MS, et al. Susceptibility contrast imaging of cerebral blood volume: human experience. Magn Reson Med 1991; 22: 293–299.

[2]   Sorensen AG, Tievsky AL, Østergaard L, Weisskoff RM, Rosen BR. Contrast agents in functional MR imaging. J Magn Reson Imaging 1997; 7: 47–55.

[2a] Østergaard L, Weisskoff R, Chesler D, Gyldensted C, Rosen B. High resolution measurement of cerebral blood flow using intravascular tracer bolus pasages. Part I: Mathematical approach and statistical analysis. Magn Reson Med 1996; 36: 715–725.

[2b] Østergaard L, Sorensen A, Kwing K, Weisskoff R, Gyldensted C, Rosen B. High resolution measurement of cerebral blood flow using intravascular tracer bolus pasages. Part II: Experimental comparison and preliminary results. Magn Reson Med 1996; 36: 726–736.

[3]   Villringer A, Rosen BR, Belliveau JW, Ackerman JL, Lauffer RB, Buxton RB, Chao YS, Wedeen VJ, Brady TJ. Dynamic imaging with lanthanide chelates in normal brain: contrast due to magnetic susceptibility effects. Magn Reson Med 1988; 6: 164–174.

[4]   Grubb RL, Raichle ME, Eichling JO, Ter-Pogossian MM. The effects of changes in $PaCO_2$ on cerebral blood volume, blood flow, and vascular mean transit time. Stroke 1974; 5: 630–639.

[5]   Powers WJ. Cerebral hemodynamics in ischemic cerebrovascular disease. Ann Neurol 1991; 29: 231–240.

[6]   Powers WJ, Grubb RL, Raichle ME. Physiological responses to focal cerebral ischemia in humans. Ann Neurol 1984; 16: 546–552.

[7]   Zaharchuk G, Mandeville JB, Bogdonov Jr AA, Weissleder R, Rosen BR, Marota JJA. Cerebrovascular dynamics of autoregulation and hypotension: an MRI study of CBF and changes in total and microvascular cerebral blood volume during hemorrhagic hypotension. Stroke 1999; 30(10): 2197–2203; discussion 2204–5 (Oct.).

[8]   Sorensen AG, Copen W, Østergaard L, Buonanno F, Gonzalez R, Rordorf G, Rosen B, Schwamm L, Weisskoff R, Koroshetz W. Hyperacute stroke: Simultaneous measurement of relative cerebral blood volume, relative cerebral blood flow, and mean tissue transit time. Radiology 1999; 210: 519–527.

[9]   Weisskoff R, Chesler D, Boxerman J, Rosen B. Pitfalls in MR measurement of tissue blood flow with intravascular tracers: which mean transit time? Magn Reson Med 1993; 29: 553–558.

[10] Belliveau J, Rosen B, Kantor H, Rzedzian R, Kennedy D, McKinstry R, Vevea J, Cohen M, Pykett I, Brady T. Functional cerebral imaging by susceptibility-contrast NMR. Magn Reson Med 1990; 14: 538–546.

[11] Rosen B, Belliveau J, Buchbinder B, Kwong K, Poorka L, Fisel R, Weisskoff R, Neuder M, Aronnen H, Cohen M, Hopkins A, Brady T. Contrast agents and cerebral hemodynamics. Magn Reson Med 1991; 19: 285–292.

[12] Rosen B, Belliveau J, Vevea J, Brady T. Perfusion imaging with NMR contrast agents. Magn Reson Med 1990; 14: 249–266.

[13] Belliveau J, Kennedy D, McKinstry R, Buchbinder B, Weisskoff R, Cohen M, Vevea J, Brady T, Rosen B. Functional mapping of the human visual cortex. Science 1991; 254: 716–719.

[14] Fisel CR, Ackerman JL, Buxton RB, Garrido L, Belliveau JW, Rosen BR, Brady TJ. MR contrast due to microscopically heterogeneous magnetic susceptibility: numerical simulations and applications to cerebral physiology. Magn Reson Med 1991; 17: 336–347.

[15] Majumdar S, Zoghbi SS, Gore JC. Regional differences in rat brain displayed by fast MRI with superparamagnetic contrast agents. Magn Reson Imaging 1988; 6: 611–615.

[16] Henkelman RM, Hardy PA. Contrast in the presence of magnetic particulates. Seventh Annual Meeting of the Society of Magnetic Resonance Imaging, Los Angeles, CA 1989.

[17] Boxerman JL, Hamberg LM, Rosen BR, Weisskoff RM. MR contrast due to intravascular magnetic susceptibility perturbations. Magn Reson Med 1995; 34: 555–566.

[18] Ogawa S, Lee T, Kay A, Tank D. Brain magnetic resonance imaging with contrast dependent on blood oxygenation. Proc Natl Acad Sci 1990; 87: 9868–9872.

[19] Ogawa S, Lee TM. Magnetic resonance imaging of blood vessels at high fields: in vivo and in vitro measurements and image simulation. Magn Reson Med 1990; 16: 9–18.

[20] Ogawa S, Lee TM, Nayak AS, Glynn P. Oxygenation-sensitive contrast in magnetic resonance image of rodent brain at high magnetic fields. Magn Reson Med 1990; 14: 68–78.

[21] Thulborn KR, Waterton JC, Matthews PM, Radda GK. Oxygenation dependence of the transverse relaxation time of water protons in whole blood at high field. Biochim Biophys Acta 1982; 714: 265–270.

[22] Zaharchuk G, Bogdanov Jr, AA, Marota JJ, Shimizu-Sasamata M, Weisskoff RM, Kwong KK, Jenkins BG, Weissleder R, Rosen BR. Continuous assessment of perfusion by tagging including volume and water extraction [CAPTIVE]: a steady-state contrast agent technique for measuring blood flow, relative blood volume fraction, and the water extraction fraction. Magn Reson Med 1998; 40: 666–678.

[23] Boxerman JL, Rosen BR, Weisskoff RM. Signal-to-noise analysis of cerebral blood volume maps from dynamic NMR imaging studies. J Magn Reson Imaging 1997; 7: 528–537.

[24] Weisskoff R, Boxerman J, Sorensen A, Kulke S, Campbell T, Rosen B. Simultaneous blood volume and permeability mapping using a single Gd-based contrast in-

jection. Proceedings of the Second Meeting of the Society of Magnetic Resonance, San Francisco 1994; 279.

[25] Detre J, Subramanian V, Mitchell M, Smith D, Kobayashi A, Zaman A, Leigh J. Measurement of regional cerebral blood flow in cat brain using intracarotid ^2H_2O and ^2H NMR imaging. Magn Reson Med 1990; 14: 389–395.

[26] Williams D, Detre J, Leigh J, Koretsky A. Magnetic resonance imaging of perfusion using spin inversion of arterial water. Proc Natl Acad Sci 1992; 89: 212–216.

[27] Edelman R, Siewert B, Darby D, Thangaraj V, Nobre A, Mesulam M, Warach S. Qualitative mapping of cerebral blood flow and functional localization with echo-planar MR imaging and signal targeting with alternating radio frequency. Radiology 1994; 192: 513–520.

[28] Weisskoff R, Zuo C, Boxerman J, Rosen B. Microscopic susceptibility variation and transverse relaxation: theory and experiment. Magn Reson Med 1994; 31: 610–610.

[29] Østergaard L, Chesler DA, Weisskoff RM, Sorensen AG, Rosen BR. Modeling cerebral blood flow and flow heterogeneity from magnetic resonance residue data. J Cereb Blood Flow Metab 1999; 19: 690–699.

[30] Vogel J, Kuschinsky W. Decreased heterogeneity of capillary plasma flow in the rat whisker-barrel cortex during functional hyperemia. J Cereb Blood Flow Metab 1996; 16: 1300–1306.

[31] Kuschinsky W, Paulson OB. Capillary circulation in the brain. Cerebrovasc Brain Metab Rev 1992; 4: 261–286.

[32] Hudetz AG, Feher G, Kampine JP. Heterogeneous autoregulation of cerebrocortical capillary flow: evidence for functional thoroughfare channels? Microvasc Res 1996; 51: 131–136.

[33] Hudetz AG, Biswal BB, Feher G, Kampine JP. Effects of hypoxia and hypercapnia on capillary flow velocity in the rat cerebral cortex. Microvasc Res 1997; 54: 35–42.

[33a] Dennie J, Mandeville JB, Boxerman JL, Packard SD, Rosen BR, Weiskoff RM. NMR imaging of changes in vascular morphology due to tumor angiogenesis. Magn Reson Med 1998; 40(6): 793–799.

[34] American Heart Association. Stroke Facts 1999.

[35] Moseley ME, Cohen Y, Mintorovitch J, Chileuitt L, Shimizu H, Kucharczyk J, Wendland MF, Weinstein PR. Early detection of regional cerebral ischemia in cats: comparison of diffusion and T2 weighted MRI and spectroscopy. Magn Reson Med 1990; 14: 330–346.

[36] Gonzalez RG, Schaefer PW, Buonanno FS, Schwamm LH, Budzik RF, Rordorf G, Wang B, Sorensen AG, Koroshetz WJ. Diffusion-weighted MR imaging: diagnostic accuracy in patients imaged within 6 hours of stroke symptom onset. Radiology 1999; 210: 155–162.

[37] Warach S, Chien D, Li W, Ronthal M, Edelman RR. Fast magnetic resonance diffusion-weighted imaging of acute human stroke. Neurology 1992; 42: 1717–1723.

[38]   Warach S, Gaa J, Siewert B, Wielopolski P, Edelman R. Acute human stroke studied by whole brain echo planar diffusion-weighted magnetic resonance imaging. Ann Neurol 1995; 37: 231–241.

[39]   Davis R, Bulkley G, Traystman R. Role of oxygen free radicals in focal brain ischemia. In: Tomita M, Sawada T, Naritomi H, Heiss W-D, eds., Cerebral hyperemia and ischemia: from the standpoint of cerebral blood volume. Amsterdam: Excerpta Medica, 1988; 151–156.

[40]   Heiss W-D, Graf R. The ischemic penumbra. Current Opinion in Neurology. 1994; 7: 11–19.

[41]   Kaufmann AM, Firlik AD, Fukui MB, Wechsler LR, Jungries CA, Yonas H. Ischemic core and penumbra in human stroke [see comments]. Stroke 1999; 30: 93–99.

[42]   Karonen JO, Vanninen RL, Liu Y, Østergaard L, Kuikka JT, Nuutinen J, Vanninen EJ, Partanen PL, Vainio PA, Korhonen K, Perkio J, Roivainen R, Sivenius J, Aronen HJ. Combined diffusion and perfusion MRI with correlation to single-photon emission CT in acute ischemic stroke: ischemic penumbra predicts infarct growth. Stroke 1999; 30: 1583–1590.

[43]   Symon L. The relationship between CBF, evoked potentials, and the clinical features in cerebral ischemia. Acta Neurol Scand 1980; 62: 175–190.

[44]   Tomlinson F, Anderson R, Meyer F. Acidic foci within the ischemic penumbra of the New Zealand white rabbit. Stroke 1993; 24: 2030–2040.

[45]   Furlan M, Marchal M, Viader F, Derlon J-M, Baron J-C. Spontaneous neurological recovery after stroke and the fate of the ischemic penumbra. Ann Neurol 1996; 40: 216–226.

[46]   Marchal G, Beaudouin V, Rioux P, de la Sayette V, Le Doze F, Viader F, Derlon JM, Baron JC. Prolonged persistence of substantial volumes of potentially viable brain tissue after stroke: a correlative PET-CT study with voxel-based data analysis [see comments]. Stroke 1996; 27: 599–606.

[47]   Rosner G, Heiss W. Survival of cortical neurons as a function of residual flow and duration of ischemia. J Cereb Blood Flow Metab 1983; 3: S393–394.

[48]   Inoue T, Kato H, Araki T, Kogure K. Emphasized selective vulnerability after repeated nonlethal cerebral ischemic insults in rats. Stroke 1992; 23: 739–745.

[49]   Tievsky A, Gonzalez RG, Lev MH, et al. Correlation of DWI/MTT mismatch and MRA/CTA in acute stroke. 36th Annual Meeting of the Amerian Society of Neuroradiology, Philadelphia, PA 1998.

[50]   Warach S, Wielopolski P, Edelman RR. Identification and characterization of the ischemic penumbra of acute human stroke using echo-planar diffusion and perfusion imaging. Twelfth Annual Meeting of the Society of Magnetic Resonance in Medicine, New York 1993; 249.

[51]   Baird AE, Benfield A, Schlaug G, Siewert B, Lovblad K-O, Edelman RR, Warach S. Enlargement of human cerebral ischemic lesion volumes measured by diffusion-weighted magnetic resonance imaging. Ann Neurol 1997; 41: 581–589.

[52] Lovblad KO, Baird AE, Schlaug G, Benfield A, Siewert B, Voetsch B, Connor A, Burzynski C, Edelman RR, Warach S. Ischemic lesion volumes in acute stroke by diffusion-weighted magnetic resonance imaging correlate with clinical outcome. Ann Neurol 1997; 42: 164–170.

[53] Schwamm LH, Koroshetz WJ, Sorensen AG, Wang B, Copen WA, Budzik R, Rordorf G, Buonanno FS, Schaefer PW, Gonzalez RG. Time course of lesion development in patients with acute stroke: serial diffusion- and hemodynamic-weighted magnetic resonance imaging. Stroke 1998; 29: 2268–2276.

[54] Lutsep HL, Albers GW, De Crespigny A, Kamat GN, Marks MP, Moseley ME. Clinical utility of diffusion-weighted magnetic resonance imaging in the assessment of ischemic stroke. Ann Neurol 1997; 41: 574–580.

[55] Tong DC, Yenari MA, Albers GW, O'Brien M, Marks MP, Moseley ME. Correlation of perfusion and diffusion weighted MRI with NIH SS score in acute ischemic stroke. Neurology 1998; 50: 864–870.

[56] Warach S, Dashe JF, Edelman RR. Clinical outcome in ischemic stroke predicted by early diffusion-weighted and perfusion magnetic resonance imaging: a preliminary analysis. J Cereb Blood Flow Metab 1996; 16: 53–59.

[57] Hatazawa J, Shimosegawa E, Toyoshima H, Ardekani BA, Suzuki A, Okudera T, Miura Y. Cerebral blood volume in acute brain infarction: A combined study with dynamic susceptibility contrast MRI and 99 mTc-HMPAO-SPECT. Stroke 1999; 30: 800–806.

[58] Kluytmans M, van der Grond J, Folkers PJ, Mali WP, Viergever MA. Differentiation of gray matter and white matter perfusion in patients with unilateral internal carotid artery occlusion. J Magn Reson Imaging 1998; 8: 767–774.

[59] Wolpert SM, Bruckmann H, Greenlee R, Wechsler L, Pessin MS, del Zoppo GJ. Neuroradiologic evaluation of patients with acute stroke treated with recombinant tissue plasminogen activator. The rt-PA Acute Stroke Study Group. Am J Neuroradiol 1993; 14: 3–13.

[60] Wolf PA, Belanger AJ, D'Agostino RB. Management of risk factors. Neurologic Clinics 1992; 10: 177–191.

[61] Hier DB, Foulkes MA, Swiontoniowski M, Sacco RL, Gorelick PB, Mohr JP, Price TR, Wolf PA. Stroke recurrence within two years after ischemic infarction. Stroke 1991; 22: 155–161.

[62] Crosby D, Simonson T, Fisher D, Weyenberg C, Ehrhardt J, Michalson L, Sato Y, Rezai K, Yuh W. Echo-planar MR imaging: correlation of intracranial perfusion-sensitive imaging with cerebral angiography. Second Meeting, Society of Magnetic Resonance, San Francisco 1994; 277.

[63] Tsuchiya K, Inaoka S, Mizutani Y, Hachiya J. Echo-planar perfusion MR of moyamoya disease. Am J Neuroradiol 1998; 19: 211–216.

[64] Tzika AA, Robertson RL, Barnes PD, Vajapeyam S, Burrows PE, Treves ST, Scott RM. Childhood moyamoya disease: hemodynamic MRI. Pediatr Radiol 1997; 27: 727–735.

[65] Sato N, Bronen RA, Sze G, Kawamura Y, Coughlin W, Putman CM, Spencer DD. Postoperative changes in the brain: MR imaging findings in patients without neoplasms. Radiology 1997; 204: 839 – 846.

[66] Johnson PC, Hunt SJ, Drayer BP. Human cerebral gliomas: correlation of post-mortem MR imaging and neuropathologic findings. Radiology 1989; 170: 211 – 217.

[67] Earnest FT, Kelly PJ, Scheithauer BW, Kall BA, Cascino TL, Ehman RL, Forbes GS, Axley PL. Cerebral astrocytomas: histopathologic correlation of MR and CT contrast enhancement with stereotactic biopsy. Radiology 1988; 166: 823 – 827.

[68] DiChiro G. Positron emission tomography [^{18}F] fluorodeoxyglucose in brain tumors: a powerful diagnostic and prognostic tool. Investigative Radiology 1986; 22: 360 – 371.

[69] Alavi J, Alavi A, Charoluk J, et al. Positron emission tomography in patients with glioma: A predictor of prognosis. Cancer 1988; 62: 1074 – 1078.

[70] Yoshii Y, Moritake T, Suzuki K, Fujita K, Nose T, Satou M. Cerebral radiation necrosis with accumulation of thallium 201 on single-photon emission CT. Am J Neuroradiol 1996; 17: 1773 – 1776.

[71] Ricci PE, Karis JP, Heiserman JE, Fram EK, Bice AN, Drayer BP. Differentiating recurrent tumor from radiation necrosis: time for re-evaluation of positron emission tomography? Am J Neuroradiol 1998; 19: 407 – 413.

[72] Weidner N, Semple JP, Welch WR, Folkman J. Tumor angiogenesis and metastasis-correlation in invasive breast carcinoma. New Engl J Med 1991; 324: 1 – 8.

[73] Weidner N, Carroll PR, Flax J, Blumenfeld W, Folkman J. Tumor angiogenesis correlates with metastasis in invasive prostate carcinoma. Am J Pathol 1993; 143: 401 – 409.

[74] Leon SP, Folkerth RD, Black PM. Microvessel density is a prognostic indicator for patients with astroglial brain tumors. Cancer 1996; 77: 362 – 372.

[75] Okunieff P, Dols S, Lee J, Singer S, Vaupel P, Neuringer LJ, Beshah K. Angiogenesis determines blood flow, metabolism, growth rate and ATPase kinetics of tumors growing in an irradiated bed: ^{31}P and ^{2}H nuclear magnetic resonance studies. Cancer Res 1991; 51: 3289 – 3295.

[76] Ariza A, Fernandez LA, Inagami T, Kim JH, Manuelidis EE. Renin in glioblastoma multiforme and its role in neovascularization. Am J Clin Pathol 1988; 90: 437 – 441.

[77] Zagzag D, Miller DC, Sato Y, Rifkin DB, Burstein DE. Immunohistochemical localization of basic fibroblast growth factor in astrocytomas. Cancer Res 1990; 50: 7393 – 7398.

[78] Plate KH, Breier G, Farrell CL, Risau W. Platelet-derived growth factor receptor-beta is induced during tumor development and upregulated during tumor progression in endothelial cells in human gliomas. Laboratory Investigation 1992; 67: 529 – 534.

[79] Russel DC, Rubinstein LJ. Pathology of Tumours of the Nervous System. Arnold, London 1989.

[80]   Brem S. The role of vascular proliferation in the growth of brain tumors. Clin Neurosurg 1976; 23: 440–453.

[81]   Plate KH, Breier G, Weich HA, Risau W. Vascular endothelial growth factor is a potential tumour angiogenesis factor in human gliomas in vivo. Nature 1992; 359: 845–848.

[82]   Burger PC, Vogel FS, Green SB, Strike TA. Glioblastoma multiforme and anaplastic astrocytoma: pathologic criteria and prognostic implications. Cancer 1985; 56: 1106–1111.

[83]   Aronen H, Gazit I, Louis D, Buchbinder B, Pardo F, Weisskoff R, Harsh G, Cosgrove G, Halpern E, Hochberg F, Rosen B. Cerebral blood volume maps of gliomas: comparison with tumor grade and histologic findings. Radiology 1994; 191: 41–51.

[84]   Aronen H, Gazit I, Pardo F, Nitschke M, Jiang H, Cohen M, Hochberg F, Fischman A, Campbell T, Brady T, Rosen B. Multislice MRI CBV imaging of brain tumors: a comparison with PET studies. Proceedings of the Twelfth Annual Scientific Meeting, New York 1993; 485.

[85]   Hao D, DiFrancesco LM, Brasher PM, deMetz C, Fulton DS, DeAngelis LM, Forsyth PA. Is primary CNS lymphoma really becoming more common? A population-based study of incidence, clinicopathological features and outcomes in Alberta from 1975 to 1996. Ann Oncol 1999; 10: 65–70.

[86]   Daumas-Duport C, Scheithauer B, O'Fallon J, Kelly P. Grading of astrocytomas. A simple and reproducible method. Cancer 1988; 62: 2152–2165.

[87]   Ellison D, Love S, Chimelli L, Harding B, Lowe J, Roberts G, Vinters H. Neuropathology. Mosby 1998.

[88]   Morantz RA. Radiation therapy in the treatment of cerebral astrocytoma. Neurosurgery 1987; 20: 975–982.

[89]   Chamberlain MC, Murovic JA, Levin VA. Absence of contrast enhancement on CT brain scans of patients with supratentorial malignant gliomas. Neurology 1988; 38: 1371–1374.

[90]   Coffey RJ, Lunsford LD, Taylor FH. Survival after stereotactic biopsy of malignant gliomas. Neurosurgery 1988; 22: 465–473.

[91]   Greenberg MS. Handbook of Neurosurgery. Greenberg Graphics, Lakeland, FL 1994; 856.

[92]   Delbeke D, Meyerowitz C, Lapidus RL, Maciunas RJ, Jennings MT, Moots PL, Kessler RM. Optimal cutoff levels of F-18 fluorodeoxyglucose uptake in the differentiation of low-grade from high-grade brain tumors with PET. Radiology 1995; 195: 47–52.

[93]   Di Chiro G, DeLaPaz R, Brooks R, Sokoloff L, Kornblith P, Smith B, Patronas N, Kufta C, Kessler R, Johnston G, Manning R, Wolf A. Glucose utilization of cerebral gliomas measured by [^{18}F]-fluorodeoxyglucose and positron emission tomography. Neurology 1982; 32: 1323–1329.

[94]   Aronen HJ, Glass J, Pardo FS, Belliveau JW, Gruber ML, Buchbinder BR, Gazit IE, Linggood RM, Fischman AJ, Rosen BR, et al. Echo-planar MR cerebral blood volume mapping of gliomas. Clinical utility. Acta Radiologica 1995; 36: 520–528.

[95] Knopp EA, Johnson G, Golfinos JG, et al. Echo-planar perfusion imaging in the evaluation and management of patients with intracranial neoplasms: The NYU experience. 83rd Scientific Assembly and Annual Meeting of the Radiological Society of North America, Chicago, IL 1997.

[96] Lev MH, Barest G, Schaefer P, et al. Is high grade glioma present? The diagnostic value of magnetic resonance relative cerebral blood volume imaging of intra-cranial neoplasia. 83rd Scientific Assembly and Annual Meeting of the Radio-logical Society of North America, Chicago, 1997.

[97] Lev MH, Schaefer PW, Barest GD, et al. Radiation necrosis or glioma recurrence? Magnetic resonance relative cerebral blood volume imaging in proton beam treated patients. 82nd Scientific Assembly and Annual Meeting of the Radiological Society of North America, Chicago, IL 1997.

[98] Sorensen AG, Kulke SM, Weisskoff RM, Boxerman JL, Buchbinder BR, Rosen BR. Investigation of cerebral hemodynamics with sprodiamide [Dy-DTPA-BMA] and functional magnetic resonance imaging. American Society of Neuroradiology Annual Meeting, Nashville, TN 1994; 237.

[99] Lev MH, Kwong KK, Rabinov J, et al. The clinical utility of perfusion-weighted echo-planar IRSE functional MR imaging in the evaluation of intracranial neo-plasms. 81st Scientific Assembly and Annual Meeting of the Radiological Society of North America, Chicago, IL 1995.

[100] Lev MH, Barest G, Kwong K, et al. Arterial spin labeled perfusion MRI of native and treated human brain tumors: preliminary comparison with dynamic contrast en-hanced rCBV and PET-FDG imaging. 36th Annual Meeting of the American Society of Neuroradiology, Philadelphia, PA 1998.

[101] Østergaard L, Hochberg FH, Rabinov JD, Sorensen AG, Lev M, Kim L, Weisskoff RM, Gonzalez RG, Gyldensted C, Rosen BR. Early changes measured by magnetic resonance imaging in cerebral blood flow, blood volume, and blood-brain barrier permeability following dexamethasone treatment in patients with brain tumors. J Neurosurg 1999; 90: 300–305.

[102] Wong ET, Jackson EF, Hess KR, Schomer DF, Hazle JD, Kyritsis AP, Jaeckle KA, Yung WK, Levin VA, Leeds NE. Correlation between dynamic MRI and outcome in patients with malignant gliomas. Neurology 1998; 50: 777–781.

[103] Sugahara T, Korogi Y, Shigematsu Y, Hirai T, Ikushima I, Liang L, Ushio Y, Takahashi M. Perfusion-sensitive MRI of cerebral lymphomas: a preliminary report. J Comput Assist Tomogr 1999; 23: 232–237.

[104] Ernst TM, Chang L, Witt MD, Aronow HA, Cornford ME, Walot I, Goldberg MA. Cerebral toxoplasmosis and lymphoma in AIDS: perfusion MR imaging experience in 13 patients. Radiology 1998; 208: 663–669.

[105] Lev MH, Schaeffer P, Sorensen AG, et al. Clinical utility of functional MRI of cerebral blood volume in the evaluation of intracranial tumors. 33rd Annual meeting of the American Society of Neuroradiology, Chicago, IL 1995.

[106] Scherer HJ. The forms of growth in gliomas and their practical significance. Brain 1940; 63: 1–35.

[107] Sorensen AG, Kulke S, Aronen H, Weisskoff RM, Rischman A, Hochberg FH, Pardo FS, Harsh G, Rosen BR. Relative cerebral blood volume maps can distinguish tumor recurrence from radiation necrosis. 33rd Annual Meeting of the American Society of Neuroradiology, Chicago, IL 1995.

[108] Wenz F, Rempp K, Hess T, Debus J, Brix G, Engenhart R, Knopp MV, van Kaick G, Wannenmacher M. Effect of radiation on blood volume in low-grade astrocytomas and normal brain tissue: quantification with dynamic susceptibility contrast MR imaging. Am J Roentgenol 1996; 166: 187–193.

[109] Wenz F, Rempp K, Brix G, Knopp MV, Guckel F, Hess T, van Kaick G. Age dependency of the regional cerebral blood volume [rCBV] measured with dynamic suscepti- bility contrast MR imaging [DSC]. Magn Reson Imaging 1996; 14: 157–162.

[110] Rempp KA, Brix G, Wenz FRBC, Gückel F, Lorenz WJ. Quantification of regional cerebral blood flow and volume with dynamic susceptibility contrast-enhanced MR imaging. Radiology 1994; 193: 637–641.

[111] Herholz K, Perani D, Salmon E, Franck G, Fazio F, Heiss W D, Comar D. Com- parability of FDG PET studies in probable Alzheimer's disease. J Nucl Med 1993; 34: 1460–1466.

[112] Tohgi H, Yonezawa H, Takahashi S, Sato N, Kato E, Kudo M, Hatano K, Sasaki T. Cerebral blood flow and oxygen metabolism in senile dementia of Alzheimer's type and vascular dementia with deep white matter changes. Neuroradiology 1998; 40: 131–137.

[113] Gonzalez RG, Fischman AJ, Guimaraes AR, Carr CA, Stern CE, Halpern EF, Growdon JH, Rosen BR. Functional MR in the evaluation of dementia: correlation of abnor- mal dynamic cerebral blood volume measurements with changes in cerebral metabolism on positron emission tomography with fludeoxyglucose F 18. Am J Neuroradiol 1995; 16: 1763–1770.

[114] Harris GJ, Lewis RF, Satlin A, English CD, Scott TM, Yurgelun-Todd DA, Renshaw PF. Dynamic susceptibility contrast MR imaging of regional cerebral blood volume in Alzheimer disease: a promising alternative to nuclear medicine. Am J Neuroradiol 1998; 19: 1727–1732.

[115] Harris GJ, Lewis RF, Satlin A, English CD, Scott TM, Yurgelun-Todd DA, Renshaw PF. Dynamic susceptibility contrast MRI of regional cerebral blood volume in Alz- heimer's disease. Am J Psychiatry 1996; 153: 721–724.

[116] Neff KW, Gueckel F, Schwartz A, et al. Assessment of cerebral hemodynamics in subcortical vascular encephalopathy by using dynamic susceptibility contrast- enhanced MR imaging. 82nd Scientific Assembly and Annual Meeting of the Radiological Society of North America, Chicago, IL 1996.

[117] Essig M, Wenz F, Knopp M, et al. Cerebral blood flow in patients with dementia syndrome. 82nd Scientific Assembly and Annual Meeting of the Radiological Society of North America, Chicago, IL 1996.

[118] Stern CE, Corkin S, Gonzalez RG, Guimaraes AR, Baker JR, Jennings PJ, Carr CA, Sugiura RM, Vedantham V, Rosen BR. The hippocampal formation participates in novel picture encoding: evidence from functional magnetic resonance imaging. Proc Natl Acad Sci USA 1996; 93: 8660–8665.

[119] American Heart Association. Causes of Death, 1996. From www.americanheart.org/statistics.

[120] Cutrer FM, Sorensen AG, Weisskoff RM, Østergaard L, Sanchez del Rio M, Lee EJ, Rosen BR, Moskowitz MA. Perfusion-weighted imaging defects during spontaneous migrainous aura. Ann Neurol 1998; 43: 25–31.

[121] Warach S, Levin JM, Schomer DL, Holman BL, Edelman RR. Hyperperfusion of ictal seizure focus demonstrated by MR perfusion imaging. Am J Neuroradiol 1994; 15: 965–968.

[122] Jackson GD, Connelly A, Cross JH, Gordon I, Gadian DG. Functional magnetic resonance imaging of focal seizures. Neurology 1994; 44: 850–856.

[123] Falconer MA. Mesial temporal (Ammon's horn) sclerosis as a common cause of epilepsy. Etiology, treatment, and prevention. Lancet 1974; ii: 767–770.

[124] Wu RH, Bruening R, Noachtar S, Arnold S, Berchtenbreiter C, Bartenstein P, Drzezga A, Tatsch K, Reiser M. MR measurement of regional relative cerebral blood volume in epilepsy. J Magn Reson Imaging 1999; 9: 435–440.

[125] Tracey I, Hamberg LM, Guimaraes AR, Hunter G, Chang I, Navia BA, Gonzalez RG. Increased cerebral blood volume in HIV-positive patients detected by functional MRI. Neurology 1998; 50: 1821–1826.

[126] Streeter CC, Ciraulo DA, Harris GJ, Kaufman MJ, Lewis RF, Knapp CM, Ciraulo AM, Maas LC, Ungeheuer M, Szulewski S, Renshaw PF. Functional magnetic resonance imaging of alprazolam-induced changes in humans with familial alcoholism. Psychiatry Res 1998; 82: 69–82.

[127] Rostrup E, Larsson HB, Toft PB, Garde K, Ring PB, Henriksen O. Susceptibility contrast imaging of CO_2-induced changes in the blood volume of the human brain. Acta Radiologica 1996; 37: 813–822.

[128] Kaufman MJ, Levin JM, Maas LC, Rose SL, Lukas SE, Mendelson JH, Cohen BM, Renshaw PF. Cocaine decreases relative cerebral blood volume in humans: a dynamic susceptibility contrast magnetic resonance imaging study. Psychopharmacology [Berl] 1998; 138: 76–81.

[129] Li KL, Suojanen JN. Cocaine-induced changes in time course of regional cerebral blood volume and transit time as determined by dynamic MR imaging. J Magn Reson Imaging 1995; 5: 715–718.

[130] Berthezene Y, Nighoghossian N, Damien J, Derex L, Trouillas P, Froment JC. Effects of thalamic hemorrhage on cortical hemodynamic parameters assessed by perfusion MR imaging: preliminary report. J Neurol Sci 1998; 157: 67–72.

[131] Tzika AA, Massoth RJ, Ball Jr, WS, Majumdar S, Dunn RS, Kirks DR. Cerebral perfusion in children: detection with dynamic contrast-enhanced T2*-weighted MR images. Radiology 1993; 187: 449–458.

[132] Cohen BM, Yurgelun-Todd D, English CD, Renshaw PF. Abnormalities of regional distribution of cerebral vasculature in schizophrenia detected by dynamic susceptibility contrast MRI. Am J Psychiatry 1995; 152: 1801 – 1803.

[133] Petrella JR, DeCarli C, Dagli M, Grandin CB, Duyn JH, Frank JA, Hoffman EA, Theodore WH. Age-related vasodilatory response to acetazolamide challenge in healthy adults: a dynamic contrast-enhanced MR study. Am J Neuroradiol 1998; 19: 39 – 44.

[134] Nighoghossian N, Berthezene Y, Meyer R, Cinotti L, Adeleine P, Philippon B, Froment JC, Trouillas P. Assessment of cerebrovascular reactivity by dynamic susceptibility contrast-enhanced MR imaging. J Neurol Sci 1997; 149: 171 – 176.

[135] Petrella JR, DeCarli C, Dagli M, Duyn JH, Grandin CB, Frank JA, Hoffman EA, Theodore WH. Assessment of whole-brain vasodilatory capacity with acetazolamide challenge at 1.5 T using dynamic contrast imaging with frequency-shifted burst. Am J Neuroradiol 1997; 18: 1153 – 1161.

[136] Chen YC, Galpern WR, Brownell AL, Matthews RT, Bogdanov M, Isacson O, Keltner JR, Beal MF, Rosen BR, Jenkins BG. Detection of dopaminergic neurotransmitter activity using pharmacologic MRI: correlation with PET, microdialysis, and behavioral data. Magn Reson Med 1997; 38; 389 – 398.

[137] Zaharchuk G, Ledden PJ, Kwong KK, Reese TG, Rosen BR, Wald LL. Multislice perfusion and perfusion territory imaging in humans with a separate label and image coils. Magn Reson Med 1999; 41: 1093 – 1098.

[138] Sorensen AG, Rosen B. Functional MRI of the brain. In: Atlas Scott W., ed. Magnetic Resonance Inaging of the Brain and Spine. Philadelphia: Lippencott-Raven, 1996; 1501 – 1545.

[139] Portions of this section are modified from [138] with permission.

Index